The Social Context of AIDS

AMERICAN SOCIOLOGICAL ASSOCIATION PRESIDENTIAL SERIES

Volumes in this series are edited by successive presidents of the American Sociological Association and are based upon sessions at the Annual Meeting of the organization. Volumes in this series are listed below.

JAMES F. SHORT, Jr.
The Social Fabric: Dimensions and Issues (1986)

MATILDA WHITE RILEY
in association with
BETTINA J. HUBER and BETH B. HESS
**Social Structures and Human Lives:
Social Change and the Life Course, Volume 1** (1988)

MATILDA WHITE RILEY
Sociological Lives: Social Change and the Life Course, Volume 2 (1989)

MELVIN L. KOHN
Cross-National Research in Sociology (1989)

HERBERT J. GANS
Sociology in America (1990)

JOAN HUBER
Macro-Micro Linkage in Sociology (1991)

JOAN HUBER and BETH E. SCHNEIDER
The Social Context of AIDS (1992)

The above volumes are available from Sage Publications.

PETER M. BLAU
Approaches to the Study of Social Structure (1975, out of print)

LEWIS A. COSER and OTTO N. LARSEN
The Uses of Controversy in Sociology (1976, out of print)

J. MILTON YINGER
Major Social Issues: A Multidisciplinary View (1978, out of print)

AMOS H. HAWLEY
Societal Growth: Processes and Implications (1979, out of print)

HUBERT M. BLALOCK
Sociological Theory and Research: A Critical Approach (1980, out of print)

ALICE S. ROSSI
Gender and the Life Course (1985, Aldine Publishing Co.)

KAI ERIKSON and STEVEN PETER VALLAS
The Nature of Work: Sociological Perspectives (1990, Yale University Press)

Joan Huber
Beth E. Schneider
editors

The
Social
Context
of
AIDS

American Sociological Association Presidential Series

SAGE PUBLICATIONS
The International Professional Publishers
Newbury Park   London   New Delhi

Copyright © 1992 by Sage Publications, Inc.

For information address:

SAGE Publications, Inc.
2455 Teller Road
Newbury Park, California 91320

SAGE Publications Ltd.
6 Bonhill Street
London EC2A 4PU
United Kingdom

SAGE Publications India Pvt. Ltd.
M-32 Market
Greater Kailash I
New Delhi 110 048 India

Printed in the United States of America

Library of Congress Cataloging-in-Publication Data

Main entry under title:

The Social context of AIDS / edited by Joan Huber and Beth E.
   Schneider.
       p.   cm. — (American Sociological Association Presidential
   series)
    Includes bibliographical references and index.
    ISBN 0-8039-4329-6. — ISBN 0-8039-4330-X (pbk.)
    1. AIDS (Disease)—Social aspects.   I. Huber, Joan, 1925-
II. Schneider, Beth.   III. Series.
   RC607.A26S629   1991
   306.4′61—dc20   91-7433
                                                                    CIP

FIRST PRINTING, 1992

Sage Production Editor: Diane S. Foster

Contents

About the Authors

BARRY D. ADAM is Professor of Sociology at the University of Windsor and author of *The Survival of Domination* and *The Rise of a Gay and Lesbian Movement*. He is a cofounder and past president of the AIDS Committee of Windsor and is currently researching the impact of HIV upon personal and family relationships.

STEPHEN CRYSTAL (Ph.D.) is Director, AIDS Research Group; Chair, Division on Aging; and Associate Research Professor, Institute for Health, Health Care Policy and Aging Research, Rutgers University. His writings on social policy range from aging to homelessness. His AIDS research began at the University of California, San Diego, where he was Chief, Division of Health Care Sciences, School of Medicine, and has continued at Rutgers with surveys of persons with HIV illness aimed at understanding interrelationships among health services use, social support, and other dimensions of the HIV "illness career." He is Principal Investigator of "Health Care Costs and Utilization in AIDS Home Care," funded by the Agency for Health Care Policy and Research.

RICHARD CURTIS is Adjunct Assistant Professor of Anthropology at John Jay College of Criminal Justice and Senior Research Associate at the Vera Institute of Justice. He currently is directing an ethnographic study of New York City's Tactical Narcotics Team for Vera Institute. He is also ethnographic director at Narcotic and Drug Research, Inc., working on a study of social factors and HIV risk.

DON C. DES JARLAIS (Ph.D.) is Director of Research for the Chemical Dependency Institute at Beth Israel Medical Center, Deputy Director for AIDS Research with Narcotic and Drug Research, Inc., a Visiting Professor of Psychology at Columbia University, and Professor of Community Medicine at Mount Sinai's Department of Community Medicine. A leader in the fields of AIDS and intravenous drug use over the last six years, he has published over 50 articles on the topics. He was the plenary speaker on intravenous drug use and AIDS at the Third and Fourth International Conferences on AIDS and has served as consultant to various institutions, including the Centers for Disease Control, the National Institute on Drug

Abuse, the National Academy of Sciences, and the World Health Organization. He is a member of the National Commission on Acquired Immune Deficiency Syndrome.

RHODA ESTEP (Ph.D.) is Associate Professor in the Department of Sociology, California State University, Stanislaus. Her research interests include sexuality, mass media, and drug use. She teaches research methods, medical sociology, mental health, and social welfare.

SAMUEL R. FRIEDMAN (Ph.D.) is Principal Investigator at Narcotic and Drug Research, Inc., on a number of research projects on the sociology and epidemiology of HIV infection and its prevention. His publications on AIDS and IV drug use include papers on HIV epidemiology and the social and behavioral causes of risk behavior and risk reduction. His past work has included research on social movements and labor activism. He is a past member of the Board of Directors of the Society for the Study of Social Problems, past Chair of its Labor Studies Division, and past Co-Chair of the Marxist section of the American Sociological Association. He received his Ph.D. in sociology from the University of Michigan. He also is a published poet.

JENNIFER HAM received a B.A. in cultural anthropology in 1984 from the University of Vermont, Burlington, with a focus on cross-cultural women's studies. She continued her academic training at the University of California, Berkeley, receiving an M.A. in public health in 1989 in the Department of Behavioral Sciences. In addition to research conducted on the psychosocial factors underlying AIDS risk among female partners of intravenous drug users, her counseling and research experience includes domestic violence, substance abuse, reproductive health, and sexually transmitted diseases. She currently lives in San Francisco and works as an editor at a medical communication firm.

JOAN HUBER taught at Notre Dame and at the University of Illinois, Urbana-Champaign. She currently is Dean of the College of Social and Behavioral Sciences at Ohio State University. She was President of the American Sociological Association in 1989 and is Chair of the Committee on Women's Employment and Related Issues for the National Research Council. Her research interests are in gender stratification.

MARGUERITE JACKSON is Director of the Medical Center Epidemiology Unit and Assistant Clinical Professor of Community Medicine, University of California, San Diego. She is also a Ph.D. student in its Department of Sociology. She publishes and consults widely about hospital epidemiology and about patient and health care worker risks for infection. She has worked with the HIV epidemic since its beginning, including chairing the San Diego County Subcommittee for the governor's AIDS Leadership Committee. Her doctoral research is part of a Teaching Nursing Home Project funded by the National Institute on Aging.

DAVID R. KOVACS (M.Ed., M.S.) is serving his third term as President of AIDS Project/Hartford. He is a founding member of the Connecticut AIDS Action Council and does public speaking about AIDS issues. He currently is facilitating educational/therapeutic seminars for HIV-infected individuals in the Hartford area. He teaches socially and emotionally maladjusted students at a local public high school.

MARTIN P. LEVINE is Associate Professor of Sociology at Florida Atlantic University and a Research Associate at Memorial Sloan-Kettering Cancer Center, New York. He helped found and lead both the Sociologists' AIDS Network and the Lesbian and Gay Caucus and was an adviser to the Presidential Commission on the Human Immunodeficiency Virus Epidemic and the National Academy of Sciences' Panel on Monitoring the Social Impact of the AIDS Epidemic. He edited the anthology *Gay Men: The Sociology of Male Homosexuality* and has published widely on the sociology of AIDS, sexuality, and homosexuality. In addition, he has been a volunteer at the Body Positive of New York and Gay Men's Health Crisis.

TOBY MAROTTA (M.A.T., M.P.A., Ph.D.) is the author of *Sons of Harvard* and *The Politics of Homosexuality*. Since 1973, he has been conducting ethnographic research in sexual subcultures. His specialty is the study of homosexual behavior in upper-class and underclass milieus. An independent scholar, he currently is affiliated with the Institute for Scientific Analysis in San Francisco.

ALAN NEAIGUS received his Ph.D. in Sociology from the University of California, Los Angeles. He has done research on urban policy issues and worked on the New York City AIDS Task force, projecting the health care needs of people with AIDS. He is a Project Director at Narcotic and Drug Research, Inc., where he has investigated factors associated with risk reduction in intravenous drug users. Currently, he is doing research on the role of drug injectors' social networks in the transmission and prevention of HIV.

REBECCA L. ROBBINS (M.A.) is completing her Ph.D. in clinical psychology at California School of Professional Psychology, Berkeley/Alameda. Her research interests are in the area of the psychosocial impact of AIDS on the lives of women and her dissertation is on self-efficacy and AIDS risk behavior among female sexual partners of intravenous drug users.

BETH E. SCHNEIDER is Associate Professor of Sociology and Women's Studies at the University of California, Santa Barbara. Her research on sexuality at work and on lesbians has appeared in *Work and Occupations, Sociological Perspectives, Gender & Society,* and in many other chapters and articles. Her writing about AIDS has been primarily about gender and AIDS with special attention to women with AIDS. With Nancy Stoller Shaw, she currently is coediting a volume on women's place in the AIDS crisis. She served as the past Chair of the Sexual Behavior Section, Society for the Study of Social Problems, and the Sociologists' Gay and Lesbian Caucus. She currently is Co-Chair of the board of the AIDS Counseling and Assistance Program of Santa Barbara County and the Lesbian and Gay Resource Center.

MICHAEL L. SCHWALBE is Assistant Professor of Sociology at North Carolina State University. He received his Ph.D. from Washington State University in 1984. His interests are in the social psychology of the self-concept, gender socialization, and moral problem solving. Currently, he is studying processes of self-change in the contexts of creative work and intimate relationships.

KAROLYNN SIEGEL (Ph.D.) is Director of Social Work Research at Memorial Sloan-Kettering Cancer Center and Associate Professor of Sociology in Public Health at Cornell University Medical College. She has been the recipient of grants from the National Institute of Mental Health, the National Cancer Institute, the American Cancer Society, and various private foundations. She has numerous publications in the fields of AIDS, psychosocial adaptation to illness, childhood bereavement, and cancer survivorship.

BARBARA G. SOSNOWITZ (M.S.W., M.A.) is Associate Professor of Social Work and Sociology at Central Connecticut State University. She directs the undergraduate social work program. She became involved in the local AIDS project in 1985 and was instrumental in setting up intake services and group support as well as volunteer training. She was one of the founders of the very successful Greater Hartford AIDS Collaborative. She currently is doing research on the social construction of AIDS and the perception of risk among college freshmen.

CLIFFORD L. STAPLES is Assistant Professor of Sociology at the University of North Dakota. He received his Ph.D. from Washington State University in 1985. His interest is in how the self is shaped by and reproduces social inequalities. His current work focuses on the social construction of masculine identity and the role of self-evaluation in legitimating stratification.

MERYL SUFIAN (Ph.D.) is Co-Principal Investigator at Narcotic and Drug Research, Inc. on research projects related to HIV prevention. She is the author and coauthor of several papers on HIV and ethnicity and on HIV and risk reduction. She has been conducting research in the field of medical sociology for several years. She received her Ph.D. from the City University of New York Graduate School.

DAN WALDORF (M.A.) is Research Sociologist and Senior Research Scientist at the Institute for Scientific Analysis in San Francisco. He has worked in the substance abuse field for 23 years and only recently in AIDS-related work. He was Principal Investigator for the study on male hustlers and call men and is currently directing two other studies: "The Condom Use of Male Prostitutes" and "Crack Sales, Gangs and Violence."

LAURIE WERMUTH has spent the past several years as a member of the research faculty at the University of California, San Francisco. Her main area of study there has been AIDS risk among women sexual partners of intravenous drug users. In fall 1990, she became a faculty member of the Department of Sociology and Social Work at California State University, Chico.

Editors' Foreword

This volume is the result of a partnership between Beth E. Schneider and Joan Huber over the last three years. In 1988 when Huber was president-elect of the American Sociological Association, she asked Beth Schneider to serve on the program committee for the annual meeting. With the encouragement of the Sociologists' AIDS Network, of which Schneider was (and is) a member, the program committee selected "AIDS" as a second theme of the 1989 annual meeting in San Francisco. This meeting site was particularly appropriate for such a theme because San Francisco had probably gone further than any other American city in putting together an organizational response to the disease. Schneider was instrumental in the organization of the plenary, a thematic session, several regular section sessions, a forum with San Francisco AIDS activists, and a teaching workshop.

This book is the outcome of activities at those meetings. Huber and Schneider agreed that there should be a second volume for the Presidential Series that Sage publishes. Schneider, the acknowledged AIDS expert, would lead the way in planning the volume and carrying out the tasks that had to be done to bring the volume to completion. She worked with the authors on their papers, wrote the introduction, the glossary, and contributed a chapter herself. Huber provided a second reading of all the manuscripts and copyedited final drafts. Both read page proofs.

The actual division of labor was that which had been planned. Huber's name appears first as editor only because she was president of the American Sociological Association in 1989 and this volume is part of the Sage Presidential Series.

—Joan Huber
Beth E. Schneider

Introduction

In the 10 years since AIDS has been identified as a distinct clinical syndrome, sociologists have been very active in research and teaching about AIDS. Most of the authors represented in this volume are members of the Sociologists' AIDS Network, a group of activists, educators, and researchers—all sociologists—who meet yearly to provide an effective intellectual forum and network for those working on AIDS across the United States. Each of the scholars published here is in one way or another working on AIDS in his or her local community or campus. Many do this work as part of their research or teaching positions; others are volunteers. Some are engaged in both scholarship and political struggle around AIDS. With a newsletter, a directory of members and their research interests, sessions at annual meetings of the American Sociological Association and the Society for the Study of Social Problems as well as regional associations, and a bibliography of course syllabi on AIDS, the Sociologists' AIDS Network has sustained individual scholars across the country, supplying support and information while generating an interest group within the field advocating the continued presence of research on AIDS in the discipline's journals and public gatherings.

The materials in this volume are organized to highlight the kinds of directions sociological research has taken in approaching the problem of AIDS. The first part, consisting of two chapters, by Adam and Schneider, offers different, but parallel, conceptual frameworks from which research on the social context, impact, and consequences of AIDS may be conducted. In the second part, sociologists grapple with the social context and dynamics of risky behavior of self-identified gay men, women who are partners of intravenous drug users, and male prostitutes. In the last part, the four contributions provide analyses of the social context of treatment of persons with AIDS and public policy.

Each chapter is a revision of a paper presented during the 1989 Annual Meeting of the American Sociological Association held that August in San Francisco. During those meetings, as a result of the program committee's endorsement of a proposal from the Sociologists' AIDS Network, AIDS was given special attention for the first time at the professional meetings. In addition to a plenary on AIDS conducted in a large ballroom draped with selected memorial banners from the Names Project Quilt, sessions at those meetings included "San Francisco Responds to AIDS," at which local organizers and activists shared their work with sociologists; a teaching workshop; a session on "AIDS and the Family;" and two general sessions on the social context of AIDS.

For the profession, this was a major and public commitment to the study of AIDS given that organizationally little had been done earlier. Though many sociologists had published in public health, medical, and policy outlets, the peer-reviewed sociology journals have, for the most part, not offered research on AIDS until the end of the 1980s. One exception has been the *Journal of Health and Social Behavior,* an ASA publication that has included intermittent pieces about AIDS since 1987. Although specialized articles about AIDS began appearing in the psychological literature in 1984, it was not until 1987 that the *American Sociologist* published a forum about the need for a research agenda, with three sociologists—Nancy Stoller Shaw, Alice S. Rossi, and Karolynn Siegel—responding to a position paper by Richard A. Berk, "Anticipating the Social Consequences of AIDS." Other sociology journals—*Social Problems, Qualitative Sociology,* and *California Sociologist*—put out special issues in 1990. Neither of the two journals considered most mainstream—*American Sociological Review* and *American Journal of Sociology*—has yet published any articles addressing AIDS in any context.

This book demonstrates multiple sociological approaches to the AIDS epidemic. Given the chapters' unique origin, the book is necessarily an incomplete account of the current sociological work on the AIDS epidemic. The essays, taken together, raise important, as yet unanswered questions demanding further sociological discussion and research. Although the Adam and Schneider chapters explicitly set forth research agendas, each of the other pieces sets forth additional research questions. A concluding section of the introduction includes some additional directions for research on AIDS in the 1990s.

THE SOCIAL CONTEXT OF AIDS

The chapters in Part I of the volume offer a broad overview of the research on AIDS, pointing out neglected ways of seeing the problem of AIDS and topics for further examination. Each is strongly influenced by a particular conceptual approach. The chapter by Adam argues for a sociology *for* HIV-infected persons. The Schneider chapter calls for the use of a feminist perspective in understanding AIDS, one that takes seriously the intersection of race, class, and gender relations no matter who or what is studied. Each of these efforts outlines programs of research that attempt to chart theoretically informed directions for sociological investigation and analysis for the next 5 to 10 years.

In the first chapter, "Sociology and People Living with AIDS," Adam advocates strongly for research from the perspective of oppressed or subordinate groups rather than from the perspective of those who dominate cultural discourse and political and social institutions. In taking the point of view of persons living with AIDS, he notes that the study of AIDS, like all social problems research, must confront questions of who the research is for and to what end it will be put.

With an approach that makes the institution the observed rather than the observer, Adam's chapter provides a unified set of questions touching on the political economy of AIDS and the means through which persons living with HIV infection may be empowered. Whether raising questions about the ways AIDS information is produced and disseminated, or how medical and social services are distributed, or the manner in which the state has responded to AIDS, Adam's chapter stands alone in this volume in calling for comparative, historical work and putting AIDS into a global context.

In "AIDS and Class, Gender, and Race Relations," Schneider argues for, and attempts to put forward, a feminist framework that considers the relations of race, class, and gender at the heart of any analysis of the social consequences of HIV infection. She notes that these interconnected interpersonal and structural relations have and still do frame the development of AIDS as a social problem, structure its social consequences, and change as the society organizes to deal with this disease.

To illustrate these points, Schneider examines five areas of research: AIDS and its impact on men (the demographic group most affected by HIV infection), the consequences of HIV disease for women, the responses of racial and ethnic communities to AIDS, political mobilization by affected groups, and issues in social control and public policy.

Neither Adam nor Schneider directly addresses at any length the question of sociological method in studying AIDS, though each clearly raises methodological and epistemological concerns. How an issue is studied will determine the kinds of questions that may be asked and who and what may benefit from its answers. However, the work in the next two parts does demonstrate some of the uses to which sociological methods and theoretical frameworks may be employed to understand the social context of AIDS prevention, treatment, and policy.

THE SOCIAL CONTEXT
OF RISKY BEHAVIOR

Public health education is a difficult process. The need to speak to established and deeply felt emotions and values, already demonstrated in efforts to alter patterns of smoking and drinking, has been patently obvious in dealing with AIDS. Social scientists have begun to make contributions to these efforts through the application of health promotion models and behavior change protocols; psychologists and social psychologists have been in the forefront of these efforts to change individual behavior. Yet, as the contributions of the following three chapters make clear, sociologically driven analyses, particularly of the seemingly intractable aspects of education, reveal the political, cultural, and emotional context and parameters of risky behavior.

The social context of risky sexual behavior aptly describes the empirical work in the second section. In the most narrow terms, the issue addressed by this work is how to reduce the risk of HIV infection. These chapters emphasize that the substantive study of AIDS prevention has centered on three unique groups: gay men, partners of intravenous drug users, and male prostitutes. The chapters vary in attention to individual-versus group-level dimensions to account for changes in sexual behavior. Each provides findings from ongoing research projects and suggestions for further research or program development. But, in addition to the important practical implications, each piece starkly highlights the complexity of sexuality revealed through the lens of AIDS prevention. Each illustrates the need for a sociology of risky sexual behavior that uses the best insights of several sociological subfields: emotions, medicine, sexuality, social networks, and politics.

There is evidence of considerable change in the sexual practices and cultural expectations of gay men in the last decade. Condoms now are typically considered effective means to prevent the spread of HIV and their use has been increasingly deemed appropriate and acceptable. In "Unprotected Sex: Understanding Gay Men's Participation," Levine and Siegel raise a crucial, surprisingly unstudied question: What are the motives of self-identified gay men for engaging in unprotected anal or oral intercourse—that is, how is the persistence of unsafe activity explained by that portion of gay men who either sporadically or regularly engage in it?

Using Scott and Lyman's concept of "accounts," Levine and Siegel examine 124 interviews with gay men in New York City for explanations of their unprotected sexual encounters. Whether the men justified their behavior by challenging the public health model of risky behavior or by invoking highly traditional notions of "extenuating circumstances" that serve to excuse problematic sex, both kinds of accounts illustrate the power and ambiguity of sexual interaction.

Similar issues emerge in studying women and AIDS. By 1989, women had become the fastest growing category of persons diagnosed with AIDS. This pattern is expected to continue in the 1990s. In "Women Don't Wear Condoms: AIDS Risk Among Sexual Partners of IV Drug Users," Wermuth, Ham, and Robbins examine one such group, the women who are partners of intravenous-drug-using men, to reveal the implicit and explicit gender and economic dynamics underlying the potential for change in sexual interaction and behavior among heterosexual couples, particularly concerning the adoption of the use of condoms.

Critical of the individualistic and cognitive social psychological models often used to make sense of health behavior change, the authors analyze their data in terms of the five strategies devised by their 77 interviewees to reduce their uncertainty and to increase their control over risk of HIV transmission. Like the gay men discussed in the Levine and Siegel chapter, these women were highly knowledgeable about AIDS and were concerned about their risk, but few of the women reported their partners ever using condoms.

Recognizing the implications of these findings for alterations to the public health approach, which so consistently ignores discussions of power between partners but instead focuses on partners' talking about sex and the use of condoms, Wermuth and her colleagues strongly suggest that "communication skills" are insufficient. Consistent with Adam, they direct attention to the interactional nature of sex; consistent with Schneider, they call for attention to the dynamics of emotional and economic dependency as well as class and race variation in sexual practice.

The need to deal with the prevention of the spread of HIV infection forced the recognition that men who have sex with men are a wide-ranging and diverse population. In "Sexual Behavior of Male Prostitutes," Estep, Waldorf, and Marotta focus on two types of male prostitutes in the San Francisco Bay Area, delineate and account for the safe and unsafe behavior patterns of each, and offer a number of suggestions for reducing the spread of HIV among men who are prostitutes and their partners. In an analysis quite different than that of Levine and Siegel, these researchers use multiple regression statistical procedures to demonstrate that drug use, knowing someone who has died of AIDS, and number of partners served by a male prostitute are the factors that most clearly predict unsafe behavior in these two groups.

As the three studies in this part suggest, it is rare to find ethnographic research that studies prevention in action: how people actually talk to each other and convince, argue, and negotiate with one another. Access to actual encounters is quite limited; applicability of lab findings to everyday life is problematic.

THE SOCIAL CONTEXT
OF TREATMENT AND POLICY

Treatment of persons with AIDS and governmental policy occur in a particular social context that frames the available options for public action. Among the most prominent features of the social context of treatment and policy around AIDS in the United States is a punitive rather than a public health approach to drug use, a particularistic rather than a universalistic health care system, and a stigmatized rather than tolerant attitude toward homosexuality.

Each chapter in this last part makes a direct contribution to some distinct policy-related question. In turn, the chapters address working with intravenous drug users on prevention programs, support systems for AIDS caregivers, HIV-antibody testing and discrimination, and consequences of medical diagnoses and Centers for Disease Control definitions of AIDS on qualification for social benefits. As these chapters demonstrate, although neither medical ethicists nor legal scholars, social scientists have an important role in highlighting the processes involved in balancing individual and public rights.

Intravenous drug use constitutes the second most frequent means through which the human immunodeficiency virus is transmitted in the United States. Over the years, social science researchers in New York City and San Francisco have been actively involved with programs providing AIDS prevention education to intravenous drug users. There have been considerable decreases in the rate of risky drug-use practices.

Friedman, Sufian, Curtis, Neaigus, and Des Jarlais, in "Organizing Drug Users Against AIDS," report on an organizing project intended to generate new means through which to intervene with drug users to reduce the transmission of AIDS. Unlike the studies of risky behavior in the previous section, which focus primarily on individual behavior, this project, a planned intervention by a drug research group and an ex-users' program, is concerned with creating vehicles for collective behavior through the development of organizations for and by drug users. They found that it was possible for outsiders to organize drug users, that even somewhat loose organization was instrumental in reducing risky user behavior, but that the formation of indigenous organizations among practicing drug users was quite difficult. Friedman and his colleagues elaborate on the problems of organizing drug users and related problems, many of which, like limited supplies of bleach, have little to do with population characteristics as such. The authors suggest tentatively but provocatively that, in further efforts to organize drug users, neither ex-users nor drug treatment personnel be employed.

Throughout the course of the epidemic, informal mechanisms of care, typically initially organized by people with AIDS themselves, have provided the main sources of support to persons with AIDS (PWAs). Informal caregiving, though now considered the best kind of care, was a necessary consequence of the stigma of AIDS as an infectious and fatal illness, of the fear and loathing toward gay men, and of the limits of resource allocation during the Reagan presidency.

In "From Burying to Caring: Family AIDS Support Groups," Sosnowitz and Kovacs look closely at nonprofessional caregivers in the lives of persons with AIDS, comparing them with others who attend to the chronically and terminally ill. The authors, working at a community-based organization developed explicitly to deal with the problem of AIDS in Hartford, Connecticut, were themselves instrumental in encouraging the formation of support groups for caregivers and facilitated the meetings. Noting that research on the impact of an illness on the family or persons in charge of care is still minimal, the authors focus their research report on the workings of a support group for caregivers and the processes through which the group members deal with their own concerns, fears, and feelings while sustaining this crucial aspect of the caring system.

The need for public education to prevent the spread of HIV has been acknowledged throughout much of the last decade; less often is education cited as a vehicle that may affect levels of tolerance toward people living with HIV infection. Little evidence existed until recently of the need to make systematic, empirical sense of the kinds of conflicts pervasive in matters of public health policy between an individual's interest and liberty and the sense of the public good. In "Forced Blood Testing: Role Taking, Identity, and Discrimination," Schwalbe and Staples, concerned with providing a foundation for "compassionate and fair" responses to AIDS policy issues, examine how judgments about courses of action are made. Critical of any direct application of findings from surveys on AIDS knowledge and attitudes to policy planning, they use questionnaires administered to college undergraduates to provide a Meadian social psychological and ethical analysis and discussion of the values and processes that account for judgment formation. As the authors note, "The most interesting judgments people must make about AIDS policies involve instances in which group interests conflict or moral principles clash." The factorial design approach they employed revealed that a number of social psychological and demographic factors were important in predicting discriminatory actions.

Male homophobia is given considerable attention in the discussion of their findings; the authors claim that it may "be the primary impediment to implementation of humane public policies." It is interesting that virtually every piece in this volume reveals a persistent concern with homophobia, in the social construction of AIDS, in the treatment of HIV-infected persons, or as part of the context framing the creation of public policy. Serious sociological questions remain, some suggested in the Schneider chapter, about the meaning of homophobia, its genesis, and its consequences.

Consistent with other analyses of the social construction of AIDS and the importance of language in understanding the problem of HIV infection, Crystal and Jackson in the last chapter, "Health Care and the Social Construction of AIDS: The Impact of Disease Definitions," examine the ways in which the medical definition of HIV-related disease—as AIDS, as ARC, as HIV infection—is consequential for the persons so categorized. That is, how one is designated on the continuum of HIV infection makes a difference. They note that the economic consequences of any designation would be of considerably less concern if the United States provided universal health care, benefit, and welfare systems.

Crystal and Jackson provide survey data from needs assessments conducted with people with diagnosed cases of AIDS or ARC in San Diego in the middle and end of the 1980s. In brief, the analysis of the experience of this primarily white, very well-educated, and occupationally well-situated group of homosexual men indicates clearly that economic loss is a primary concern for all, but that those with HIV infection without the

diagnosis of AIDS, even if they are very sick, suffer gr
disadvantage: less income, fewer benefits, and less access tc
nation with the seemingly more severe diagnosis brings mᵤᵣ
and, ironically, more psychological certainty. It is not surprising that the
authors call for a reevaluation of the language used by medical practitioners and media as well as a reconsideration of the governmental policy that
favors those with the presumedly more serious diagnoses.

SOME FUTURE DIRECTIONS

The range of possible research questions on the social context, social
impact, and social consequences of AIDS is great. As we noted earlier,
both chapters in Part I are veritable mines of research ideas, and each of
the other chapters suggests additional lines of work. Here, five further
topical areas are briefly outlined.

Chronicity and Ambiguity

With changes in the nature of the illness, and a move away from the
conceptualization of AIDS as an acute illness to a chronic one, many
aspects of our current understandings of the social aspects of AIDS may
need modification or serious alteration. As Sosnowitz and Kovacs suggest, "Expanding therapies and medical interventions have increased
hopes that AIDS is becoming a treatable chronic disease. The caregivers
of PWAs often find themselves in a shadowland of fearful hope." As yet,
there is scant attention to the alterations such changes in definition yield
for persons with HIV infection, for their caregivers, and for the viability
of the institutions of care. Neither have differences among persons with
AIDS, who vary widely along this dimension, been studied with regard
to the personal, interpersonal, and institutional experience.

The Emotional Care Systems

Sociologists of health have already noted the continued need for informal care providers to deal not only with the impact of AIDS but also
other illnesses, particularly those of the elderly. There is a pressing need
to make systematic sense of personal and social ramifications for the
familial and nonfamilial AIDS volunteers. Comparative examinations of
household and kinship forms and their relationship to effective informal

care are necessary. Organizationally, it is not just in San Francisco that the volunteer base is exhausted. Across the country, staff of community-based AIDS organizations report that finding volunteers is an increasing problem. In some locations, the change in clientele of persons with AIDS adds immeasurably to the problem. What will happen to the size of the pool of volunteers, and the quality of care, under these conditions? Where will new ones come from? What measures will be used by agencies and by individuals to avoid the problem of burnout?

Institutional Analyses

Sociologists are involved in research in all the institutions that have and will provide care and education to deal with aspects of the epidemic. Yet most of that research has focused on individual behavior and change. Institutional analyses remain scarce. As both Schneider and Adam suggest, there is no social organization without some impact on the lives of people with AIDS. We assume that sociologists would be interested in questions of viability and change in organizations and the personnel most dedicated to dealing with AIDS: the community-based groups, the medical facilities, the school systems, the churches. Likewise, there seems an obvious need to examine how, if at all, certain industries understood to be experiencing a dramatic loss, such as fashion and entertainment, are managing the personnel loss, the emotional trauma, and the creative change.

The Lesbian and Gay Community

For researchers interested in lesbian and gay studies, one of the more exciting ventures would be an investigation into the ways in which AIDS has or has not strengthened and altered the growth and infrastructure of the community. There certainly have been many claims that suggest both its flowering and its demise. For example, Altman (1987) suggests that AIDS is now so much part of gay men's experience as to "further isolate us from both lesbians and non-gays, while strengthening our own communal organizations." Others note, as a sign of growth, the participation of lesbians within community organizations once led by gay men. Moreover, a dire practical and sociological need exists to move away from modeling all discussion of the impact of AIDS in lesbian and gay communities on the experience of San Francisco and New York.

AIDS has made clear that gay identity and community are not grounded solely in relations of sexuality. Many theoretically driven research efforts are possible, some focusing on cultural differences in these patterns and others focusing on the processes of coming out and the ways in which AIDS has been integrated into the social experience and patterns of sexual activity of recently self-identified gay men. Finally, there is now a generation of gay men between the ages of 25 and 50 who might be labeled AIDS survivors, ones who, given the social and demographic patterns of gay life, could well have become infected but did not. A range of sociological methods might well be marshaled to specify the practical, political, and cultural meaning of surviving.

Cultural Products

With a few notable exceptions, sociologists have not been in the forefront of making sense of the cultural meanings of AIDS or in documenting the social construction of AIDS as a social problem. This is rather surprising but perhaps predictable given the propensity of most researchers to concern themselves with practical matters of prevention and policy. However, there is a constantly expanding set of cultural products (literature, novels, the Names Project Quilt) created by people who are actively engaged in a personal and/or political struggle with AIDS. Likewise, popular television media have been slow but not absent in providing day- and nighttime programming about AIDS. The cultural imagery of the ill is an important theme in historical accounts (Fee and Fox 1988); capturing the contemporary imagery has not yet been significantly approached by sociologists of culture or language.

—Beth E. Schneider
Joan Huber

REFERENCES

Altman, Dennis. 1987. *AIDS in the Mind of America*. New York: Anchor.

Fee, Elizabeth and Daniel Fox, eds. 1988. *AIDS: The Burdens of History*. Berkeley: University of California Press.

Part I
The Social Context of AIDS

1

Sociology and People
Living with AIDS

Barry D. Adam

Sociology has, with few exceptions, been a latecomer to the study of
AIDS, yet sociological paradigms and insights could have a critical role
in AIDS prevention and in the amelioration of the effects of AIDS upon
both infected and uninfected people. The slowness of the sociological
response has meant that a number of issues, where sociological expertise
could be especially useful, now have been defined and developed by a
range of researchers in epidemiology, public health, nursing, and psychology. This chapter contends that a sociological voice has much to contribute to important research issues and practical solutions to problems
presented by AIDS.

In defining such an agenda, there is no escape from the fundamental
epistemological issues raised by research on other contentious problems.
The creation of knowledge necessarily implies finding out *about* something *for* someone. The researcher, the research subject, and the research
consumer and audience are socially located, and their relationships shape
the questions posed, the data collected, and the conclusions drawn
(Barnes 1977; Mulkay 1979). Though many research reports deploy
scientific language to conceal their commitments and speak in the voice

AUTHOR'S NOTE: I would like to thank participants in the American Sociological Association workshop on researching AIDS (Miami 1989) and, in particular, John Gagnon, Martin
Levine, Beth Schneider, Nancy Shaw, Rose Weitz, Marcia Lipetz, and Rick Zimmerman for
their comments.

of an "objective," "neutral," or universal observer, they, nevertheless, betray moral positions in their discursive structures.

The critique of (often concealed) commitments in social research is now well established in a wide range of research areas, among them race relations (Ladner 1973), women's studies (Smith 1987), labor studies (Ferrarotti 1979), gay studies (Plummer 1981; Adam 1986), and social deviance (Conrad and Schneider 1980; Pfohl 1985; Cohen 1985). The classic pattern revealed by these critiques involves the application of dominant norms to the measurement of social relations among subordinate people. Their intimate relationships, attitudes, and collective actions are thereby found to be "troubled," defective, or pathological, leading to the creation of a knowledge base exploitable by agents of social control who then have warrant to administer the lives of the subordinate through therapy or incarceration. The resulting scientific images come to be used to invalidate the experiences of the oppressed and to legitimate state domination or professional control, ultimately feeding back into ideologies that blame the victim (see Adam 1978; Foucault 1980; Touraine 1988).

Existing sociological work on AIDS has not been exempt from the problems inherent in a top-down research agenda that investigates AIDS *for* state and corporate institutions and thus (by default) constructs people living with HIV infection as the "other," the object, or the problem of research. This chapter cautions sociologists to make such commitments with care and to consider an alternative research agenda for people living with HIV infection.

THE INSTITUTION AS OBSERVER

Certainly, research to answer problems identified by, for example, the health care system, the judicial system, and the insurance industry has a place in meeting the AIDS crisis. This research agenda addresses such questions as the fiscal problem that AIDS poses for health administration, problems of counting and predicting the magnitude of infection, the financial strain on the insurance industry, housing practices in prisons, and the mounting of "effective prevention programs" in schools, businesses, prisons, and the military (see Berk 1988). It tends to envision problem solving as the development of cadres of "experts" who will work with institutions, which are presumed to be benevolent and cooperative, to tutor or control the ignorant (see Berk 1987).

People at risk or suffering from HIV infection tend to be variously constructed as people "with little education, lengthy criminal histories, and weak ties to their families and larger community" (Berk 1987, p. 213), as people with "nothing to lose" and so having "disastrous consequences for social order" (Berk 1987, p. 217), as inhabitants of "marginal subcultures in society" (Messeri 1988, p. 6), or as variable-determined machines of maladaptation (Kaplan, Johnson, Bailey, and Simon 1987). The implicit model endorsed by this style of analysis is that of professional intervention into a tangle of pathology. The person with AIDS is annihilated as a subject and assigned the role of "problem."

THE INSTITUTIONS OBSERVED

Without a critical examination of its presumptions, research may start from shaky premises derived from "common sense" or conventional morality. Fortunately, recent work that examines the social construction of AIDS in society (Patton 1985; Altman 1987; Watney 1987; Fee and Fox 1988; Crimp 1988; Aggleton and Homans 1988; Aggleton, Hart, and Davies 1989; Adam 1989; Clatts and Mutchler 1989; Carter and Watney 1989) offers precautions to social scientists in defining their research problems.

AIDS has been swept into contemporary debates over the disestablishment of the nuclear family and the rights of people to take up new domestic and sexual arrangements of their own choosing (Adam 1987). The construction of AIDS "problems" inevitably takes part in larger rivalries over the "ownership" and colonization of AIDS "territory" by social movements, the professions, the media, and the state. The assignment of responsibility for the transmission and prevention of the disease occurs within moral parameters valorizing opposing positions taken over gender, sexuality, and reproduction. As with earlier conflicts over the problematization of inferiorized people, the people most directly bearing the burden, in this case of living with AIDS, are frequently "lost in the shuffle," caricatured, or spoken for. There is no privileged or omniscient vantage point from which social researchers can observe this "terrain." The conception of what and who is the "problem," and how solutions will arrive, inevitably enters into the practical arena.

The lessons from previous critiques of research on subordinated peoples suggest how a research agenda might give voice to those most affected by HIV disease, as follows.

(1) How AIDS information is produced and distributed. AIDS has a short history, having been named and given meaning only since 1981. In that period, a number of actors have sought to assimilate the syndrome into their own symbolic systems and, at times, to wield HIV infection as an instrument to accomplish a variety of goals (Adam 1989). This social construction of AIDS images has profound consequences for all aspects of public policy about the disease. It shapes state budget priorities, it places the disease among its competitors for medical research, and it defines the "worth" and moral status of its sufferers. Among the contenders for symbolic "ownership" are journalists, preachers, politicians, physicians, public health officials, gay organizations, people with AIDS coalitions, AIDS political action groups, and community-based organizations dedicated to public education and support of the afflicted. Each has its own set of interests and impact upon the generation of AIDS discourse.

To take a case in point, there is still much to be learned from study of the blockages in the information distribution system that inhibit the dissemination of practical information about how to avoid HIV transmission. Though public education to prevent transmission is often conceived as a problem of how "experts" can convince the uninformed public of the need for risk reduction, the development and propagation of practical information about HIV transmission and avoidance through "safer sex" was pioneered by grass roots organizations at a time when state agencies refused to recognize the syndrome (Altman 1987, p. 162). When state-funded mass media projects have been developed, they have been directed first to the "general population" at lowest risk of transmission, while gay, black, Hispanic, and injection-drug-using women and men have had to depend on the more meager resources of community-based organizations. In the United States and the United Kingdom, AIDS funding has been explicitly qualified by legislative bans on the "promotion" of homosexuality in printed materials.

The AIDS information system raises larger issues about the overall social organization of information production and distribution in different societies. The pattern of the spoken and the unspoken, especially in the educational system and the media with the widest reach, reveal an organization of power concerning who may speak (authoritatively) to whom. Of research interest is the social organization of impediments to the extension of knowledge about how drugs may be taken without risking HIV infection or how to have sex safely, especially when that information might reach youth and gay people. The study of the social organization of HIV information treats some of the fundamental contests of our time over who controls whose bodies and sexuality.

(2) How an AIDS folklore evolves and is integrated into everyday life. Surveys of basic AIDS knowledge now reveal a fairly high and widespread awareness of AIDS information. What is still not well understood is as follows: how AIDS knowledge is reconciled with existing stocks of knowledge, resistance to AIDS information (Nelkin 1987; Ross 1988), and disjunctures between knowledge and practice (Baldwin and Baldwin 1988).

If AIDS education programs are to be useful and effective, they must address underlying interpretive resources. The primary correlate of AIDS phobia is homophobia (Nelkin 1987; Triplet and Sugarman 1987), and AIDS phobia typically correlates with the demographic and attitudinal factors that also predict intolerance based on race and gender (Johnson 1987). This suggests there is much to be learned from the application to homophobia of research strategies that have identified the underpinnings of racism and sexism. Sociology could have a role in exploring the homophobia/AIDS phobia of such critically placed professionals as physicians and other health workers (McCarthy 1988; Kelly, St. Lawrence, Smith, Hood, and Cook 1987; Kelly and St. Lawrence 1988, p. 152), journalists, politicians, and researchers—not simply to document it but to identify underlying factors that might lead to education programs targeted at alleviating their fears and concerns.

Risk avoidance depends on perceiving oneself as possibly susceptible to infection. Sociologists ought to be particularly adept at discovering how risk is assessed among various populations. Now that a public health AIDS discourse has been developed, there is a need to examine interpretations made of it by its recipients. The widespread identification of risk of infection with "multiple partners" and being "sexual active" may create categories in which people do not recognize themselves and may encourage denial of personal risk. A good deal of mass media treatment of AIDS has constructed people with AIDS as "other" than self (Adam 1989), and heterosexuals may be particularly resistant to the AIDS prevention message by "appraising their own vulnerability based on their evaluation of how much or little they resemble their mental representation" of the "at-risk" type of person (Siegel and Gibson 1988, p. 67).

Much of the public health strategy in AIDS education is founded on a "rational man" model of health decision making in which the individual avoids potential harm when provided with relevant information. But the prevention message will become most effective only when the most salient factors entering into risk reduction practices are identified. Lay beliefs about medical causation often diverge significantly from scientific models (Warwick, Aggleton, and Homans 1988), and immediate reference groups may prove more influential in the adoption or rejection of knowledge about AIDS. An important predictor of risk reduction among injection drug users is avoidance of needle sharing by one's peer group (Friedman et al. 1987; Des Jarlais and Friedman 1988). How these decisions are made and evolve are not well understood. Peer groups are, in turn, embedded in larger community relationships and institutions that are affected or overlaid by drug distribution networks.

As well, sexual activity is always an interaction, not just an individual decision, and the introduction of condoms or other safer sex practices into sexual negotiation depends on the meanings of sexuality for its participants. The disjuncture between AIDS knowledge and the actual practice of risk reduction may be due not to inadequate information about HIV transmission but to the perceived difficulty of introducing changes into sexual interaction and the implied moral and personal messages communicated by, for example, an insistence on the use of condoms (Pollak 1988, p. 81; Chetwynd, Horn, and Kelleher 1989; Levine, Brooks, and Siegel 1989; Izazola, Basañez, Valdespino, and Sepulveda 1989). A current interest of community-based AIDS organizations is the development of "sexual negotiating skills," and, to date, there is very little social science research directly relevant to bringing this about. Resolution of these kinds of practical dilemmas also may have important implications for the maintenance of risk reduction and avoidance of relapse.

The effectiveness of AIDS education can probably be improved by taking account of the different cultural meanings of sexuality and drug use for people differentiated by gender, race, and sexual orientation, keeping in mind that even these categories require dereification. The meanings and practices of new drug users, for example, differ from those of the more experienced (Friedman and Sotheran 1989), and factors leading from nonintravenous to intravenous drug use are poorly understood.

The tendency to research gay men primarily in the epicenters of the epidemic has limited recognition of the variations among men who do have sex with men, some of whom participate in the gay world and are reached by its communication systems and others who never identify themselves as "gay" (Bennett, Chapman, and Bray 1989). Local perceptions of AIDS and of safer sex in smaller cities, towns, and rural areas need to be identified as it is likely that they diverge from those of the gay "capitals." Recent findings show a higher adherence to safer sex practices among better educated, white gay men over 25 than among less educated, younger, black, and Hispanic gay men (Richwald et al. 1988; Linn et al. 1989), suggesting a need for innovative and culturally appropriate methods for reaching the latter.

Women may find the introduction of condoms into a heterosexual interaction more difficult than do men, while heterosexual men may be recalcitrant in adopting safer sex practices due to their low sense of vulnerability to AIDS.

Finally, none of these cultural categories can be considered discrete as many people fall into more than one of them. This kind of sex research is prerequisite to understanding the fundamental issue of how sexual or drug-using norms and expectations are constructed and thus changed. Overall, AIDS cannot be treated as a monolith. Perceptions of the disease will vary by region, social class, cultural area, gender, and generation, and these variations will need to be documented to develop the most effective prevention strategies.

(3) *How medical and social services are distributed.* There is a political economy of AIDS. At the global level, where clean needles and condoms cannot be taken for granted as readily available, HIV transmission has been affected by the lack of disposable needles even in clinical settings and by the cost of prophylaxis, which is prohibitive to the very poor. Treatment by such expensive drugs as Zidovine currently reaches perhaps 10% of those with HIV infection, almost all of whom live in the First World (Hunt 1988). Poverty, by sharply limiting the employment options of a great many people, also stimulates prostitution, and many Third World sex workers (Wilson, Sibanda, Mboyi, Msimanga, and Dube 1989; Siby et al. 1989) have limited ability to enforce safer sex on customers upon whom they depend for their livelihoods.

The United States, without guarantees of health care or a social insurance "safety net" for its citizens, cultivates its own internal "Third World," which is especially vulnerable to HIV infection. Recent epidemiological research shows that, although the rate of homosexual transmission of HIV has been leveling since 1985, heterosexual transmission and transmission through needle sharing have been increasing, and this increase has been primarily among those whom William Wilson (1988) calls "the truly disadvantaged." In a period when public funds are being cut back from clinics for those who cannot otherwise afford medical services, rates of sexually transmitted disease are rising sharply in the

inner cities (Holmes 1989). People are being turned away from both STD
and drug rehabilitation clinics for lack of funds at the same time that HIV
transmission continues to rise among injection drug users, a rise that, in
New York, has now overtaken that of homosexual transmission. Understanding of HIV transmission and prevention will remain incomplete
without linkage to research on the social conditions that make injection
drug use attractive and on the chronically poor delivery of medicine to
the poor, blacks, and Hispanics when HIV infection is rising rapidly
among these groups (Fineberg 1988; DiClemente, Boyer, and Morales
1988).

The social organization of medicine is a critical element in both the
transmission and the treatment of HIV infection. Sociologists might
examine how the wave of privatization now fashionable among conservative governments in the United States, the United Kingdom, and
Canada affects medical and social services and, in turn, provides an
ideological warrant for neglect. There is more research to be done, as
well, on how the organization of health insurance as a corporate enterprise affects the availability of health insurance for those who need it
most. Though research might be directed to the problem of the insurance
industry's difficulty in making "enough" money in the face of AIDS,
research also might examine the financial plight of people with HIV
infection facing extraordinary medical bills. The United States is in many
ways unique in the infliction of unemployment, homelessness, and medical deprivation upon people with AIDS. As John Borneman (1988) points
out in his comparison of social services available in the two Berlins, many
of the most serious problems experienced by people with HIV disease in
West Germany are much diminished in the East. Where employment
rights and unemployment provisions are strong, the threat of AIDS discrimination has none of the catastrophic implications of job loss as in the
West. Where hospital care, medical consultation, and medications are
provided at nominal charge, health status no longer depends on the ability
to pay. These survival questions, which preoccupy the disadvantaged
everywhere, are rendered especially acute by the onset of chronic illness
and are necessarily a part of the AIDS story.

(4) How drug research, production, and distribution are socially organized. There is a paradoxical contrast between an apparently well-
financed and efficient drug industry—which is able to distribute illegal
drugs throughout North America, thereby accelerating HIV transmission
through needle sharing—and an apparently less effective state and corpo-

rate drug industry charged with creating and distributing treatment for HIV infection. How does the corporate organization of the pharmaceutical industry influence research? There is a widespread suspicion in the AIDS awareness movement that drug companies will not research readily available substances because there is no money to be made from them if they prove effective against AIDS (Krieger and Appleman 1986, p. 22). Zidovine, the only approved anti-HIV drug, has an astronomical price, and frequent dramatic price hikes have occurred in the last 2 years as pentamidine has moved toward approval for general use against AIDS-related pneumonia (Hunt 1988, p. 17).

The social organization of drug development and distribution merits sociological attention. Are corporate profits and state-funded grants adequate incentive for research on the full range of potential treatments for AIDS? Is the conventional scientific research process, which relies upon episodic clinical trials, sufficient to guarantee follow-through on promising treatments? There is evidence that some drugs, which have shown preliminary promise, remain "orphaned" or waylaid. Do clinical trials adequately distribute experimental drugs among people with HIV disease? There is suspicion that some groups, such as women, children, rural people, and injection drug users, may die faster due to lack of access or exclusion from clinical trials. Is the state-administered approval process for drugs, now a cautious and lengthy procedure born of the thalidomide scandal, appropriate for a disease with an exponential growth rate and high mortality? These are questions about the social organization of science and are thus sociological issues.

(5) How the state responds to AIDS. There remain a number of outstanding issues where sociological research could elucidate the likely effects of proposed policy options and provide the evidence necessary for effective programs of AIDS prevention and support. The ready-at-hand tools so often relied upon by the state are typically the law and social control measures. Just as the invention of the Wassermann test led to a wave of compulsory syphilis testing in 1935-45 (Brandt 1988, p. 369), some governments could not resist the temptation in the mid-1980s to institute expensive compulsory testing programs directed most often toward such powerless people as prisoners and immigrants and, in some instances, toward newlyweds. Systematic coercive approaches to the control of HIV infection have been most notable in Bavaria, Cuba, and South Africa, but the sporadic use of arrest against seropositive people has been widespread in other countries (Adam 1989). The effect of the

criminalization of AIDS upon public perceptions and upon existing public health programs deserves attention. While state officials debate the effectiveness of various social control programs, from criminal prosecution of HIV transmission to quarantine of "irresponsible" people by public health authorities, community-based organizations press for democratic solutions whereby people may be empowered to take control of their health and sexuality through knowledge and technique (Sears 1990). The assessment of the effectiveness of these conflicting models should be amenable to social research.

Many U.S. jurisdictions have proven reluctant or even adamant against the provision of condoms to prisoners and needle exchange programs for injection drug users, though similar initiatives have begun in Canada and Europe (Van den Hoek,van Haastrecht, and Coutinho 1989; Stimson et al. 1989). Comparison of HIV infection rates among drug users in such cities as Edinburgh and Glasgow or Detroit and New York, where needles and syringes have been readily available in one but not the other city, show that availability does have an impact upon needle sharing and thus upon infection. Yet communities remain divided over prevention strategies perceived as "encouraging" drug use, and governments similarly avoid taking responsibility for acknowledging or being seen to "encourage" sexual activity in prisons. Evaluation research of such programs is needed, as is analysis of community responses to them.

There is much to be done in documenting how people with AIDS do cope with disease in the face of law and public policy that often exacerbate the burdens associated with the disease. State and corporate health insurance plans refuse to provide benefits to domestic partners and thus fail to support the family form and support networks that provide the greatest part of everyday support to people with HIV infection. Lack of civil rights laws concerning sexual orientation and disability due to illness opens the way to discrimination, job loss, and homelessness. While AIDS education workers try to teach gay men about safer sex, sexual decision making still occurs in conditions of social opprobrium, state criminalization, and institutional antagonism to pair bonding. Though the United States, with the highest AIDS caseload in the world, might be considered a net "exporter" of the disease, immigration law excludes seropositive foreigners, resulting in several cases of incarceration and deportation of AIDS workers visiting the United States to attend AIDS conferences. The rise of perinatal transmission raises thorny issues of how the state may intervene into the reproductive choices of women. In all of these issues, social research on the effects of existing public policies could have a role in making the case for reform.

(6) *How people living with HIV infection manage illness.* Social research should contribute not only to the knowledge apparatus of the medical and social service system but to the people living with HIV infection to facilitate a culture of coping strategies, success stories, and practical knowledge for managing the disease. To date, there is little to go on in knowing how to resist and overcome the disease. There are several rationales for doing so. Psychoneuroimmunological research suggests that social support and attitude contribute to the survival chances for people with life-threatening illness (Coates, Temoshok, and Mandel 1984; Kiecolt-Glaser and Glaser 1988). This belief has led community-based organizations to offer "buddies" to people with AIDS to provide practical and emotional support. So far, very little has been done to identify the personal support networks available to people with HIV infection, the impact of illness on these networks, and their role in maintaining the quality of life of people with AIDS. "Information is needed about the quality of life of persons with AIDS, the problems which are reducing their quality of life, how they are presently coping, and what can be done to maintain a reasonable life even if their health continues to deteriorate" (Weitz 1989).

Research that permits people with AIDS to speak for themselves without too great an overlay of preconceived theory should permit an assessment of current health and social services that have affected their lives. There are, as well, a wealth of social psychological issues raised by chronic illness in general and HIV disease in particular. Exploration of the ways in which problems associated with the disease are solved in association with close family, lovers, and friends could help sketch out a "map" through unfamiliar terrain for the newly diagnosed. The research literature developed from other life-threatening and chronic illnesses, as well as (often impressionistic) accounts arising from AIDS therapy and support groups, suggests a range of interactional issues that merit in-depth exploration.

Among the biographical dilemmas faced by seropositive people and their primary groups are the impacts of seropositive status upon personal plans and identity (Nichols 1985; Catalan 1988), upon new relationships, upon pregnancy and childbearing, and upon one's sense of mortality (Kelly and St. Lawrence 1988, pp. 97, 113; Strawn 1987; Rowe, Plum, and Crossman 1988, p. 73; Schneider 1988; Tross and Hirsch 1988).

Little work has been done on the disclosure of seropositivity and its impact upon relationships among lovers, family, and friends (Frierson, Lippmann, and Johnson 1987; Robinson, Skeen, and Walters 1987; Tiblier 1987; Pearlin, Semple, and Turner 1988; Murphy and Perry 1988; Cleveland, Walters, Skeen, and Robinson 1988; Macklin 1988; Giacquinta 1989). Primary group dynamics may be disrupted by reawakened homophobia (Rowe et al. 1988), fears of shared stigma and of infection (Newmark and Taylor 1987; Wortman and Dunkel-Schetter 1979), and shifts in financial contribution and needs.

There are few, if any, spheres of life untouched by a diagnosis of HIV disease. Workplace issues include the response of employers and coworkers and the impact of job change or loss on self-esteem and financial capabilities. The decreasing control over one's life, which often is a secondary ramification of serious illness, may overshadow or complicate strictly physical problems associated with disease.

Sociology has much to say about the management of potentially discrediting information before unsympathetic audiences, and it has more to learn about the social management of physical impairment, reduced energy, time spent on treatment, or disfigurement (Strauss 1975). Intensive qualitative research is indispensable at this level to capture the unfolding dynamics of these processes. As Elliot Mishler (1986, p. 119) remarks, the research aim is to enable respondents "to be empowered . . . not only to speak in one's own voice and to tell one's own story, but to apply the understanding arrived at to action in accord with one's own interests."

CONCLUSION

Social research and state and corporate responses still tend to lag behind initiatives taken by frontline AIDS workers and community-based organizations responding to immediate needs. Social research may be more effective if done in partnership with community AIDS groups. Sociology may have a particular contribution to make in understanding the development of the AIDS awareness movement and in offering pointers on mobilizing existing neighborhood activists, black and Hispanic organizations, and as yet unorganized people such as drug users and their sex partners or bisexual men into the struggle against AIDS (see Quimby and Friedman 1989; Adam forthcoming).

Sociologists need not presume a need to impose the facts upon recalcitrant people with AIDS but can help find out what works best and communicate that to the people most interested in putting such knowledge into practice. People with HIV infection should not appear in sociological accounts as the mysterious, intractable, or pathological other. It is noteworthy that loss of control is itself a factor correlated with fatalism and a "chance orientation" toward health risks—an attitude that increases potential exposure and transmission (Price-Greathouse and Trice 1986). The role of the social scientist should be to help empower people living with HIV infection, their friends, and frontline AIDS workers with information on how best to enhance survival chances and quality of life (see Grace 1988; Crimp 1988; Aggleton and Homans 1988; Schneider 1988; Stoller Shaw 1988).

REFERENCES

Adam, Barry D. 1978. *The Survival of Domination.* New York: Elsevier/Greenwood.
———. 1986. "The Construction of a Sociological 'Homosexual' in Canadian Textbooks." *Canadian Review of Sociology and Anthropology* 23:399-411.
———. 1987. *The Rise of a Gay and Lesbian Movement.* Boston: G. K. Hall.
———. 1989. "The State, Public Policy and AIDS Discourse." *Contemporary Crises* 13: 1-14.
———. Forthcoming. "Impacts of AIDS on the Gay Community." In *The Gay and Lesbian Experience,* edited by K. Plummer. London: Routledge & Kegan Paul.
Aggleton, Peter, Graham Hart, and Peter Davies, eds. 1989. *AIDS: Social Representations, Social Practices.* London: Falmer.
Aggleton, Peter and Hilary Homans, eds. 1988. *Social Aspects of AIDS.* London: Falmer.
Altman, Dennis. 1987. *AIDS in the Mind of America.* Garden City, NY: Doubleday.
Baldwin, John and Janice Baldwin. 1988. "Factors Affecting AIDS-Related Sexual Risk-Taking Behavior Among College Students." *Journal of Sex Research* 25:181-96.
Barnes, Barry. 1977. *Interests and the Growth of Knowledge.* London: Routledge & Kegan Paul.
Bennett, G., S. Chapman, and F. Bray. 1989. "Sexual Practices and 'Beats.' "*Medical Journal of Australia* 151:309-14.
Berk, Richard. 1987. "Anticipating the Social Consequences of AIDS." *American Sociologist* 18:3.
———. ed. 1988. *The Social Impact of AIDS in the U.S.* Cambridge, MA: Abt.
Borneman, John. 1988. "AIDS in the Two Berlins." Pp. 223-26 in *AIDS: Cultural Analysis, Cultural Activism,* edited by D. Crimp. Cambridge: MIT Press.
Brandt, Allan. 1988. "AIDS in Historical Perspective." *American Journal of Public Health* 78:367-71.
Carter, Erica and Simon Watney, eds. 1989. *Taking Liberties.* London: Serpent's Tail.

Catalan, José. 1988. "Psychosocial and Neuropsychiatric Aspects of HIV Infection." *Journal of Psychosomatic Research* 32:237-48.

Chetwynd, Jane, J. Jorn, and J. Kelleher. 1989. "Safer Sex Amongst Homosexual Men." Paper presented to the Fifth International Conference on AIDS, Montreal, June.

Clatts, Michael and Kevin Mutchler, 1989. "AIDS and the Dangerous Other." *Medical Anthropology* 10:105-14.

Cleveland, Peggy, Lynda Walters, Patsy Skeen, and Bryan Robinson. 1988. "If Your Child Had AIDS . . ." *Family Relations* 37:150-53.

Coates, Thomas, Lydia Temoshok, and Jeffrey Mandel. 1984. "Psychosocial Research Is Essential to Understanding and Treating AIDS." *American Psychologist* 39:1309-14.

Cohen, Stanley. 1985. *Visions of Social Control.* Oxford: Polity.

Conrad, Peter and Joseph Schneider. 1980. *Deviance and Medicalization.* St. Louis: C. V. Mosby.

Crimp, Douglas, ed. 1988. *AIDS: Cultural Analysis, Cultural Activism.* Cambridge: MIT Press.

Des Jarlais, Don and Samuel Friedman. 1988. "The Psychology of Preventing AIDS Among Intravenous Drug Users." *American Psychologist* 43:865-70.

DiClemente, Ralph, Cherrie Boyer, and Edward Morales. 1988. "Minorities and AIDS." *American Journal of Public Health* 78:55-57.

Fee, Elizabeth and Daniel Fox, eds. 1988. *AIDS: The Burdens of History.* Berkeley: University of California Press.

Ferrarotti, Franco. 1979. *An Alternative Sociology.* New York: Irvington.

Fineberg, Harvey. 1988. "The Social Dimensions of AIDS." *Scientific American* 259: 128-34.

Foucault, Michel. 1980. *Power/Knowledge.* New York: Pantheon.

Friedman, Samuel and Jo Sotheran. 1989. "Toward a Sociology of AIDS." Paper presented to the American Sociological Association workshop on researching AIDS. Miami, May.

Friedman, Samuel, Don Des Jarlais, Jo Sotheran, Jody Garber, Henry Cohen, and Donald Smith. 1987. "AIDS and Self-Organization Among Intravenous Drug Users." *International Journal of the Addictions* 22:201.

Frierson, Robert, Steven Lippmann, and Janet Johnson. 1987. "AIDS: Psychological Stress on the Family." *Psychosomatics* 28:65-68.

Giacquinta, Barbara. 1989. "Researching the Effects of AIDS on Families." *American Journal of Hospice Care,* May/June, pp. 31-36.

Grace, Patrick. 1988. "Living with AIDS." *Radical America* 21:44-47.

Holmes, King. 1989. "HIV Infection in the Context of Changing Epidemiological Patterns of Sexually Transmitted Diseases." Plenary address to the Fifth International Conference on AIDS. Montreal, June.

Hunt, Charles. 1988. "AIDS and Capitalist Medicine." *Monthly Review* 39:11-25.

Izazola, Antonio, R. Basañez, J. Valdespino, and J. Sepulveda. 1989. "Attitudes Explaining Desertion and Non-Use of Condoms in Gay Men in Mexico." Paper presented to the Fifth International Conference on AIDS. Montreal, June.

Johnson, Stephen. 1987. "Factors Related to Intolerance to AIDS Victims." *Journal for the Scientific Study of Religion* 26:105-10.

Kaplan, Howard, Robert Johnson, Carol Bailey, and William Simon. 1987. "The Sociological Study of AIDS." *Journal of Health and Social Behavior* 28:140-57.

Kelly, Jeffrey and Janet St. Lawrence. 1988. *The AIDS Health Crisis.* New York: Plenum.

Kelly, Jeffrey, Janet St. Lawrence, Steve Smith, Harold Hood, and Donna Cook. 1987. "Stigmatization of AIDS Patients by Physicians." *American Journal of Public Health* 77:789-91.

Kiecolt-Glaser, Janice and Ronald Glaser. 1988. "Psychological Influences on Immunity." *American Psychologist* 43:892-98.

Krieger, Nancy and Rose Appleman. 1986. *The Politics of AIDS.* Oakland: Frontline.

Ladner, Joyce, ed. 1973. *The Death of White Sociology.* New York: Vintage.

Levine, Martin, C. Brooks, and K. Siegel. 1989. "Condom Usage Decisions Among Gay Men." Paper presented to the Fifth International Conference on AIDS. Montreal, June.

Linn, Lawrence et al. 1989. "Recent Sexual Behaviors Among Homosexual Men Seeking Primary Medical Care." *Archives of Internal Medicine* 149:2685.

Macklin, Eleanor. 1988. "AIDS: Implications for Families." *Family Relations* 37:141-9.

McCarthy, Paul. 1988. "Phobic Physicians." *Psychology Today* 22:16.

Messeri, Peter. 1988. "Structural Contingency Theory and the Prevention of AIDS." Paper presented to the American Sociological Association. Atlanta, August.

Mishler, Elliot. 1986. *Research Interviewing.* Cambridge, MA: Harvard University Press.

Mulkay, Michael. 1979. *Science and the Sociology of Knowledge.* London: Allen & Unwin.

Murphy, Patrice and Kathleen Perry. 1988. "Hidden Grievers." *Death Studies* 12:451-62.

Nelkin, Dorothy. 1987. "AIDS and the Social Sciences." *Reviews of Infectious Diseases* 9:980.

Newmark, Deborah and Edward Taylor. 1987. "The Family and AIDS." In *Responding to AIDS,* edited by C. Leukefeld and M. Fimbres. Silver Spring, MD: National Association of Social Workers.

Nichols, Stuart. 1985. "Psychosocial Reactions of Persons with the Acquired Immunodeficiency Syndrome." *Annals of Internal Medicine* 103:765-7.

Patton, Cindy. 1985. *Sex and Germs.* Boston: South End.

Pearlin, Leonard, Shirley Semple, and Heather Turner. 1988. "Stress of AIDS Caregiving." *Death Studies* 12:501-17.

Pfohl, Stephen. 1985. *Images of Deviance and Social Control.* New York: McGraw-Hill.

Plummer, Kenneth, ed. 1981. *The Making of the Modern Homosexual.* New York: Barnes & Noble.

Pollak, Michael. 1988. *Les homosexuels et le Sida.* Paris: Editions Métailié.

Price-Greathouse, Judith and Ashton Trice. 1986. "Chance Health-Orientation and AIDS Information Seeking." *Psychological Reports* 59:10.

Quimby, Ernest and Samuel Friedman. 1989. "Dynamics of Black Mobilization Against AIDS in New York City." *Social Problems* 36:403-15.

Richwald, Gary et al. 1988. "Sexual Activities in Bathhouses in Los Angeles Country." *Journal of Sex Research* 25:169-79.

Robinson, Bryan, Patsy Skeen, and Lynda Walters. 1987. "The AIDS Epidemic Hits Home." *Psychology Today* 21:48-52.

Ross, Michael. 1988. "Distribution of Knowledge of AIDS." *Social Science and Medicine* 27:1295-98.

Rowe, William, Gerald Plum, and Clarence Crossman. 1988. "Issues and Problems Confronting the Lovers, Families and Communities Associated With Persons With AIDS." *Journal of Social Work and Human Sexuality* 6:71-88.

Schneider, Beth. 1988. "Gender, Sexuality and AIDS." Pp. 15-36 in *The Social Impact of AIDS in the U.S.,* edited by R. Berk. Cambridge, MA: Abt.

Sears, Alan. 1990. "AIDS and the Health of Nations." Paper presented to the Canadian Sociology and Anthropology Association. Victoria, June.

Shaw, Nancy Stoller. 1988. "Preventing AIDS Among Women." *Socialist Review* 88, 4(Fall).

Siby, Tidiane, I. Thior, J. L. Sankale, A. Gueye, I. Ndoye, and S. Mboup. 1989. "Surveillance-education sanitaire des prostituées au Sénégal." Paper presented to the Fifth International Conference on AIDS. Montreal, June.

Siegel, Karolynn and William Gibson. 1988. "Barriers to the Modification of Sexual Behavior Among Heterosexuals at Risk for Acquired Immunodeficiency Syndrome." *New York State Journal of Medicine,* February, p. 66.

Smith, Dorothy. 1987. *The Everyday World as Problematic.* Toronto: University of Toronto Press.

Stimson, G. V. et al. 1989. "The Pilot Syringe Exchange Project in England and Scotland." *British Journal of Addiction* 84:1283.

Strauss, Anselm. 1975. *Chronic Illness and the Quality of Life.* St. Louis: C. V. Mosby.

Strawn, Jill. 1987. "The Psychosocial Consequences of AIDS." Pp. 126-49 in *The Person with AIDS,* edited by J. Durham and F. Cohen. New York: Springer.

Tiblier, Kay. 1987. "Intervening with Families of Young Adults with AIDS." In *Families and Life-Threatening Illness,* edited by M. Leahey and L. Wright. Springhouse, PA: Springhouse Corporation.

Touraine, Alain. 1988. *Return of the Actor.* Minneapolis: University of Minnesota Press.

Triplet, Rodney and David Sugarman. 1987. "Reactions to AIDS Victims." *Personality and Social Psychology Bulletin* 13:265-74.

Tross, Susan and Dan Hirsch. 1988. "Psychological Distress and Neuropsychological Complications of HIV Infection and AIDS." *American Psychologist* 43:929-34.

Van den Hoek, J. A., H. van Haastrecht, and R. Coutinho. 1989. "Risk Reduction Among Intravenous Drug Users in Amsterdam Under the Influence of AIDS." *American Journal of Public Health* 79:1353-57.

Warwick, Ian, Peter Aggleton, and Hilary Homans. 1988. "Young Peoples' Health Beliefs and AIDS." In *Social Aspects of AIDS,* edited by P. Aggleton and H. Homans. London: Falmer.

Watney, Simon. 1987. *Policing Desire.* London: Comedia.

Weitz, Rose. 1989. "Ideas for a Sociological Agenda on AIDS." Paper presented to the American Sociological Association Workshop on Researching AIDS. Miami, May.

Wilson, David, Babusi Sibanda, Lilian Mboyi, Sheila Msimanga, and Godwin Dube. 1989. "Health Education Among Commercial Sex Workers in Zimbabwe, Africa." Paper presented to the Fifth International Conference on AIDS. Montreal, June.

Wilson, William. 1988. *The Truly Disadvantaged.* Chicago: University of Chicago Press.

Wortman, Camille and Christine Dunkel-Schetter. 1979. "Interpersonal Relationships and Cancer." *Journal of Social Issues* 35:120-55.

2

AIDS and Class, Gender, and Race Relations

Beth E. Schneider

Relative to other social scientists, most particularly the psychologists, few sociologists have turned sustained scholarly attention to AIDS. Those who have paid attention have concentrated where the greatest need existed, focusing on some of the groups identified by epidemiologists as "high risk" and offering skills primarily to enhance prevention efforts. Others surveyed national samples on knowledge, attitudes, and behavior about AIDS, and a few have provided analyses of the changing presentation of AIDS in the media (Albert 1986).

With the possible exception of the scholarly study of sexuality, these necessary efforts tend to borrow little from, or offer little to, ongoing sociological discourse within most of the discipline. As Gagnon (1989, p. 2) has recently noted: "An HIV-control and treatment agenda may not be at all symmetric with disciplinary agenda." The published work thus far tends to focus on the individual or on "risky" behavior with little thought to the social relations of HIV transmission or to the cultural context within which those relationships occur. Despite a few early calls for social structural and institutional analyses (Berk 1987), there has been

AUTHOR'S NOTE: This chapter is based on a paper presented at the annual meetings of the American Sociological Association, August 1989, San Francisco. Thanks to Ben Bowser, Ernest Quimby, Nancy Stoller Shaw, William Vega, and Rose Weitz for conversations on race, class, and AIDS and to the work of Barry Adam, Samuel Friedman, and Martin P. Levine over the years.

rather limited attention to the institutions that have or have not mobilized; the long-term consequences for those most affected, including medical personnel, PWAs, and their communities; and the political, economic, and social impact of AIDS on specific social institutions and on urban communities.

It has been primarily historians, social commentators, and journalists who have focused on the popular media images of AIDS, provided linguistic analyses (Treichler 1988), and examined the cultural ideology of AIDS and its link to other illnesses. Unlike Brandt (1985), Altman (1987), Shilts (1987), and Sontag (1988), sociologists have, for the most part, not examined the social reactions to AIDS. Peter Conrad (1989, p. 1) recently noted: "Perhaps sociologists take the stigmatized nature of AIDS too much for granted, thus neglecting to closely examine the causes and consequences of how the social construction of AIDS affects the types of reactions it engenders."

Moreover, the early conceptualization of AIDS as a disease of gay men (presumed to be white) or of epidemiologically defined "risk groups" (IV drug users, Haitians, men having sex with men) foreclosed the recognition by virtually everyone, including sociologists, of the racial, class, and gender relations that frame the development of AIDS as a social problem, structure the social consequences of HIV infection, and change as the society organizes to deal with this new disease.

The vast majority of people with AIDS in the United States are men, a fact often taken for granted, which limits appreciation of the gendered nature of AIDS for gay and intravenous-drug-using men. Predictably, the recognition of HIV infection in women was delayed. And, despite the highly irregular targeting of a nationality—the Haitians—as a risk group early in the epidemic, recognition of race as an important factor was minimal.

A change in direction among those concerned with AIDS has occurred in the last 3 years, spurred in part by the now-publicized changing demographics of AIDS—what is euphemistically dubbed in the press "the changing face of AIDS." Now, 90% of PWAs are male, and women make up a small but increasing proportion of cases. Racial/ethnic minorities constitute 40% of the cases of AIDS in the United States: 26% are blacks, 14% are Latinos. Relative to the proportion of the total population, blacks and Latinos have an incidence of AIDS 2 or 3 times higher than whites for homosexual and bisexual males and over 20 times higher for heterosexual males (Selik, Castro and Peppaioanov 1988). Half of the cases of AIDS among blacks and Latinos occurred among heterosexual IV drug users or their sexual partners. This high frequency of AIDS cases among racial/ethnic heterosexual IV drug users results in most of the AIDS cases among black and Hispanic women (over 70%) and children (over 80%). In the last two years, the caseloads of AIDS organizations have seen an 100% increase in the proportion of African Americans, Latinos, and Native Americans.

When race, class, and gender are placed at the center of an analysis of the social consequences of HIV infection, many complex research questions and policy dilemmas emerge. Four general sociological observations concerning race, class, and gender frame this discussion. First, race, class, and gender are the three social factors most determinant of a person's health status and his or her degree of well-being. In concert, they will affect perceptions of health and illness, kinds and availability of care, modes of delivery, anticipated illnesses, and discourse and interaction patterns of doctor-patient relationships. Second, the social relations of race, class, and gender in this country are hierarchically organized, resting on and resulting in inequalities of social and political power and control over labor, resources, and services. Third, homophobia and race, class, and gender relations influence the experiences of people with AIDS, community and political reactions, the nature of institutional practice, and the dynamics of change in the society. Fourth, and finally, AIDS, as a biological and medical phenomenon of the late twentieth century, has or will have effects on the nature of homophobia and on race, class, and gender relations.

This chapter examines several areas of current and possible research in which questions about the relationship of race, class, and gender to AIDS and the social impact of these interrelated systems emerge clearly. I move from the individual to the community to the society. In the first section, I focus on the IV-drug-using and gay men with AIDS, then turn to the particular social, sexual, and reproductive problems posed for women who are HIV infected. Third, consideration is given to the racial/ethnic communities and their response to AIDS. Fourth, I raise questions for investigation related to issues of mobilization and empowerment of HIV-infected persons and their communities. Last, I touch on issues of social control and social policy.

Given the growing but still rather limited social science of AIDS (Ergas 1987), I focus on what now is known, often relying on scholarship from psychologists, social workers, and historians, sometimes relying when necessary on suggestive but often unsystematic evidence from the popular and alternative news media. I attempt to provide some sense of those issues, situational contexts, institutional spheres, and policy domains that beg for sociological efforts. I am less interested in offering answers to questions that have barely been asked than in providing questions whose answers demand attention.

It should be clear to sociologists that, when I speak of people with AIDS or HIV-infected persons, I am not talking about a uniform group but about "cultures of people with AIDS" primarily composed of peoples who have been denied the privilege of self-definition. It is not surprising then, that I continually stress the sociological exploration of the meanings actors attribute to their own conditions and situations through close qualitative studies, because as yet, there is no systematic sociological work on any group, including white gay men, that explores how that group constructs the problem of AIDS, visualizes its dangers, perceives its challenges, and acts.

MEN AND HIV INFECTION

Of the people living with AIDS in the United States, 90% are male. Most of what has been written about AIDS is focused on these men. But neither the sizable research on psychosocial issues nor the burgeoning work of researchers focused on IV drug users discusses these men as gendered persons with unique problems or unique patterns of survival.

Although conceptions of gender have changed and are not uniformly endorsed or enacted, the male as a good provider (Bernard 1981), and success at work equated with manliness, remain nearly universal. The real man obviously is heterosexual. He is a sexual initiator, and, in the pre-AIDS, 1970s version, he was always sexually ready. Being male means not seeking assistance; to get help is stigmatizing. What is the relationship of these gender expectations to the ways men act—that is, "do" gender—in an AIDS epidemic?

Gay Men

Most of the medical, psychological, and social effects of AIDS in the United States can be most clearly seen in what is written about or by gay men. With the exception of dealing with the management of sexual identity, many of the personal consequences—such as dealing with illness in the prime of life, deaths of loved ones, managing wide-ranging threats to civil liberties—necessarily affect other persons with AIDS similarly.

An examination of three social consequences to gay men—changes in sexual practices, altered interpersonal relationships, and confrontations with death—reveals the meaning and practice of gender. The gay male sexual life-style of the 1970s affirmed an ideology of sex outside of relationships and sexual adventure as a positive good. The development of a highly structured commercial, urban gay milieu occurred in a historical context of social, religious, and legal discrimination, which tends to foster internalized homophobia (Adam 1978) and is coterminous with the advent of highly political local and national communities of lesbians and gay men (Altman 1987). This combination of factors had consequences for individual identity, community activity, and sexual behavior (J. Foster 1988; Epstein 1987).

Despite evidence to the contrary, prevailing views of gay male sexual behavior denied differences among male homosexuals in sexual practice and relationship commitment (Bell and Weinberg 1978) and relied on the assumption that male sexual behavior is devoid of emotions, feelings, or community attachments. As Kayal (1986) noted, the masculinist basis of gay male culture and values resembled closely the ideology of male sexuality.

Many of the linkages between ways of doing gender in sexual relations and community interests are revealed in the changes that have and have not occurred in the sexual realm. The AIDS crisis has transformed gay male sexual practice. At the aggregate level, gay men, if sexual at all, have fewer sexual partners and less often engage in unsafe sexual practices (McKusick, Horstman, and Coates 1986; Rosen 1986). These reductions are most evident when there are high concentrations of AIDS cases and when there is a well-organized gay community that provides social support and alternative ways of being sexual (Fineberg 1988). Although the virtue of sexual adventure has been tarnished, the prospect of pleasurable sex has not.

The change in the gay men's community, which highlights social context and organization as key factors in sexual practice risk reduction, is an important challenge to all individualistic conceptions of behavioral change including those of many social psychologists. A similar process of change is occurring among IV drug users. These patterns call for the broadest sort of social network analyses to examine the impact of community and opinion leaders, role models, friends, and lovers on every group affected by AIDS to explore the paths used to communicate about and make change and the group dynamics maintaining these paths (Zimmerman 1989). In this regard, it is crucial to think sociologically about safe-sex "relapsers" and young men newly self-identified as gay.

Numerous first-person accounts of the impact of AIDS suggest that gay men, especially those situated in thriving lesbian/gay communities, have integrated the immediacy of death into daily life. This too has meant an increased appreciation of the meanings and the labor involved in nurturing and caregiving. For some gay men, an AIDS diagnosis is their first experience of getting psychological support and giving care to another (J. Foster 1988; Mandel 1986). Interrante (1987) equates his experience as the partner of a man with AIDS with the best of mothering activities: unconditional love, physical caregiving, and investment in separation. He offers a hypothesis worthy of further consideration, that dealing with death is, itself, a gendered event based in differences between men and women in their experiences of their bodies and in the birthing of children. These activities raise important questions about the social organization and management of death that go beyond what psychologists typically offer; neither are they simply questions for medical sociologists.

Finally, the experience of gay men with AIDS reveals a heightened acknowledgment of the need for support from family and friends (Macks and Turner 1986; Mandel 1986). Personal accounts indicate that gay men are more concerned than they once explicitly were with relational rather than recreational sexuality, commitment, and intimacy (Altman 1987) and that many with diagnosed cases of AIDS are entering partnerships with other men (Callen 1988). Families of gay men, like those of other PWAs, have demonstrated a spectrum of responses from outright rejection to total support (Interrante 1987; Macks and Turner 1986).

In all three of these areas, the changes that are occurring for gay men emphasize ways of doing gender typically attributed to women. Sociological analyses might be attempted on the meanings to gay men of these changes and how they have occurred. Accounts are needed for the variability in family support and the creation of kin structures of partners, friends, and children within the gay male community. No one has yet attempted important comparative work on the "returning home to die" experiences of those gay men or IV drug users who choose to do so.

These accounts are primarily by and about white gay men. Considerable effort is necessary to overcome the virtual silence of racial/ethnic gay men in their communities and the absence of these gay men in social science. The Bell and Weinberg (1978) study in San Francisco revealed some specific differences in sexual practices prior to AIDS between blacks and whites; little was known about Latinos. One recent study in

Detroit revealed that black gay men were less knowledgeable about AIDS than black IV drug users (Williams 1986). Cultural differences and racism isolate many racial/ethnic minority men from usual sources of information available to white gay men (Dawson and Thornberg 1988; DiClemente, Boyer and Morales 1988). Antihomosexual attitudes in some cultures act as barriers preventing reception of information (Peterson and Marin 1988). And many minority men have homosexual experiences but do not identify themselves as gay men; their routes to sex are numerous, and they are either simultaneously or sequentially bisexual.

The kind of community-based interventions accomplished among white gay men have been less effective with minority men; there are very few formal gay organizations in minority communities, especially outside large metropolitan areas. Such groups are only useful for those who identify themselves as homosexual. Additionally, Sabogal, Marin, Otero-Sabogal, Marin, and Perez-Stable (1987) argue that small group discussions are not likely to work for Latinos because of a strong cultural prohibition against sharing personal problems with non-family members. On the other hand, the possible roots of change may be found in the fact that activist minority lesbians and gay men are coming out in order to work on AIDS in their own black and Latino neighborhoods (Johnson, Munoz, and Pares 1988).

Male IV Drug Users

Unlike gay males, analyses of IV drug users rarely begin to touch directly on issues of gender but focus instead on a matrix of race or class factors. That intravenous drug users are men is taken for granted.

IV drug users are often characterized as alienated, antisocial, economically poor, and without social support systems and personal ties (O'Neill 1987; Z. Foster 1988). There is no doubt that institutional racism, economic marginality, powerlessness, and isolation frame their lives. The cultural stigmatization of IV drug use, and the current rhetoric linking it to the concept of a pathological underclass, diverts attention from the problems of race and results in a denial of IV drug users' links to kin and community (Des Jarlais, Friedman, and Strug 1986) and a denial of the reality of variation among users in terms of type of drug and relationship to it (ex-addict, recreational, regular, or long-term user).

Given the demographics of IV drug use, and recognizing that IV drug users are not all alike, many of these men doubtless have failed to validate their own cultural expectations for men as fathers, husbands, or sexual partners. How could it be otherwise when, for example, the status of black males between 15 and 24 years of age has not improved appreciably in the last 25 years and, in the last 10 years, has deteriorated in terms of rates of unemployment, median income, school and college attendance, homicide, and drug use? Almost half (45%) of black men do not have jobs. Drug dealing, as well as using, is a way to earn a living for economically marginal families in a capitalist society. Dealing is common in poor Hispanic New York communities (Worth and Rodriguez 1987), and the drug industry has created lucrative jobs for young black men in many urban areas across the country. Making sociological sense of these men's lives and their reactions to AIDS requires accepting the fact that drug dealing is one means to get by and to avoid failure as a man in low-income communities.

Although some commentators early in the epidemic assumed that IV drug users will "refuse to consider using safe practices" (Z. Foster 1988), there is now considerable evidence that IV drug users in many urban areas are altering their risk of contracting AIDS through changes in needle-using practices (Magura et al. 1989; Friedman et al. 1987; O'Neill 1987). Like sexual changes among gay men, IV drug users change when positive peer support exists to resist pressures to share needles and when the material means are readily available to use drugs differently (Magura et al. 1989). Though there has also been a sizable increase in the numbers of IV drug users attempting to enter treatment, research is necessary on the racial and class patterns of this movement to cease drug use (Des Jarlais and Friedman 1988) as well as on geographic, racial, and ethnic differences in patterns of needle sharing and use of "shooting galleries."

Other research topics in the area of drug abuse are particularly urgent for the next few years. First, adolescents in many racial and cultural communities are at risk for HIV infection, at least in part because the desire for peer acceptance leads to drugs and sex. In New York City, AIDS has not become a primary reason to avoid drug injections (Des Jarlais, Casriel, and Friedman 1988); the newer, less-well-integrated users are also least informed about safe use of needles (Des Jarlais and Friedman 1988). Will new users learn about HIV transmission from formal prevention programs or through the drug subculture? To answer this narrow question, a larger ethnographic investigation seems appropriate to delineate the ways in which the IV-drug-use subculture, with its structured interpersonal networks of "running partners," is making adjustments to the facts of AIDS or introducing new users (women, adolescents) to changed ways of drug use. It is not surprising that studies on the subjectivity of IV-drug-user PWAs or HIV-infected persons are scarce, though the research of Friedman and his associates (1987) on efforts to organize IV drug users suggests considerable potential for the development of solidarity and self-defense in this population.

Second, crack—cheaper than heroin and a purported sexual stimulant—threatens to become an additional, indirect source of HIV transmission (Bowser 1988). Studies similar to Bowser's in San Francisco on the social organization of crack use are needed for a variety of ethnic communities and other cities.

Although changes have occurred in the ways drugs are administered, sexual transmission is a continuing issue (Des Jarlais and Friedman 1988). The negotiation of change in any heterosexual relation is complicated. Particularly, but certainly not exclusively, in black and Latino communities, many men have sex with men but do not identify themselves as homosexual or even bisexual (Worth and Rodriguez 1987; Hammonds 1987). Peterson and Marin (1988) note that many black and Latin drug users do not disclose their antibody status to their female partners for fear of rejection and loss of support. Many female partners of men from Latino communities may not be aware of the sexual practices of the men with whom they associate given the cultural prescriptions against such discussion as well as homosexual activity. Moreover, they see the men as superior to them, will not talk about sex because "good women" do not, and defer to men in decision making related to sex. Being prepared for sex may violate not only church dictate but their sense of virtuous womanhood (Worth and Rodriguez 1987). The women may be emotionally and economically dependent; threats of physical coercion may silence them; and the negotiations around condom use may be psychologically uncomfortable (Peterson and Marin 1988). It has proven easier to introduce condoms into casual sexual relations where little emotional investment exists than in long-standing, committed relations (Des Jarlais and Friedman 1988).

In looking at heterosexual sex through the lens of race and class, we observe how absolutely necessary research is to understand what makes change in the sexual realm. As the history of sexually transmitted diseases makes clear, neither information nor fear alone fosters change in behavior (Brandt 1985; Fineberg 1988; Ergas 1987). Thus far, it has been only the organized community of gay men that has developed educational models that take full account of the meanings connected to sexuality in efforts to transform it (Altman 1987). Within the context of unique racial/ethnic communities, the complexity of this relationship is compounded by sexism and heterosexism. Though we do not, as yet, know what they are, the meanings of safer sex must vary at the very least by gender and between racial/ethnic groups.

HIV-INFECTED WOMEN

Women with AIDS do not fit into the male AIDS profiles because neither of these adequately addresses some of the central physiological or sociopolitical differences between women and men and neither situates these women in their own unique historical and material conditions. Without attention to the intersection of gender, class, and race (Collins 1986), it is next to impossible to understand the particular situation of the vast majority of HIV-infected women.

Nationally, drug use accounts for 50% of the female AIDS cases. Though regional differences exist, the proportion of women getting AIDS from male sexual partners has steadily increased since 1982 (Shaw 1988). Of all women with AIDS, 70% are black and Latino, and, of the total, over half reside in the New York/New Jersey metropolitan area and Florida. In New York City, AIDS is now the major cause of death in women aged 25 to 29 years.

HIV-infected women do not constitute a self-conscious, politically active community. Most of the women currently at highest risk or with AIDS are least likely to have access to adequate medical care or health insurance. The public, to the extent that it has awareness of these women, no doubt can easily scapegoat female intravenous drug users and poor women of color. Women are conventionally blamed for their pregnancies, abortions, sexually transmitted diseases, and prostitution (Schneider 1988; Shaw and Paleo 1986).

In addition, the life conditions and social psychological stresses for women (especially those with children) differ markedly from those of most men, especially white homosexual men about whom most research concerning AIDS has been undertaken and for whom most services concerning AIDS are organized. And all social psychological dimensions that have an impact on stress (coping strategies, role strain, life events, and social support) are theoretically constructed differently for racial/ethnic groups (Kaplan 1983). Even medically, the women with AIDS are different. HIV-infected women continue to be misdiagnosed. On the aggregate, women are dying faster than men. For the first time, and only in the name of newborns, pregnant women in 1989 were enrolled in certain drug trials to which previously they had been excluded ("Pregnant Women" 1989).

Three areas of sociological research are very much needed that put these women at the center: research on female IV drug users, on AIDS and its impact on mothering, and on women's efforts to transform sexual relationships. The research that exists on female IV drug users is quite limited. Until this decade, women as IV drug users were disregarded because they did not fit into the "typescripts" of the drug addict (Robins 1980). These women often are still invisible in the research on IV drug users and AIDS. The literature on heroin use and women (Worth and Rodriguez 1987; Rosenbaum 1981) suggests that the women are different than men in that they come later to drug use, enter the heroin culture through introduction by a man, have larger habits, may rely on prostitution to support their drug use, and have children for whom they are caring. Some, but not all, of these women experience a conflict between their efforts to attain heroin and their mothering (Moore and Devitt 1989; Rosenbaum 1981).

Reliance on studies of women using heroin are insufficient to grapple with some additional or new factors such as the impact of membership in gangs on women users (Moore and Devitt 1989) or the use of methadone or crack on women's lives (Bowser 1988). We still need to know more about how women become involved in drug use, especially in racial/ethnic communities. Factors that lead to the use of needle sharing among young women are not clear.

A second and broader avenue of investigation lies in delineating the unique quality of these women's lives as they confront the impact of AIDS on the emotional, psychological, and social aspects of their mothering. Virtually all women with AIDS are mothers; 80% of the children with AIDS acquired it through their mothers who have AIDS or are HIV infected. And numerous unanswered issues remain surrounding pediatric AIDS (Schneider 1988; National Academy of Sciences 1986).

Women, but especially those who may be HIV infected, have been urged to postpone pregnancy until researchers address medical quandaries regarding pregnancy and pediatric AIDS. But a decision to forgo pregnancy or terminate a pregnancy typically is not made lightly for most women. Women, whatever their cultural heritage, confront issues in the AIDS epidemic about control over their reproductive futures and sexual desires, the meaning of children for them, and values concerning abortion. Situational opportunities often determine women's decisions about childbearing. These issues have varying significance and impact among women of different class, ethnic, and racial backgrounds.

Black teenagers, for example, are more sexually active than whites and are less likely to use contraception and abortion, and the black proportion of births to single women is higher (Zelnick and Kanter 1980). These facts, in part, reflect historically specific views of the value of children and black community support of single motherhood (O'Connell 1980; Thompson 1980) and, in part, reflect the interlocking structures of race and class oppression. Though there are class differences, it is through motherhood that most Latinas affirm their status as women (Andrade 1982; Moore and Devitt 1989). The limited research on female heroin users (mostly black) reveals that their children and motherhood are their singular claim to worthiness (Rosenbaum 1981). Hence, any understanding of motherhood in these women's lives must touch on the choices available to them within opportunity structures, their material conditions, and their perceptions of the possibilities for themselves and their children.

Sociological research has thus far revealed little about the impact of the introduction of AIDS on their lives. Some of the losses and changes are similar to those of gay men. But, as mothers and as women of color, their relationship to their children and wider kin system is a prominent issue. For HIV-infected women, their activities as primary parent are invariably transformed. Family patterns may be disrupted. Who will care for the mother and her children? What does care mean given the relative lack of resources? How does the kinship network help or hinder? And what does she feel about herself and her options? How does she decide what is best for her children in the event she dies when confronted with the fact that there are an estimated 50,000 to 100,000 children who are not sick but have been orphaned by AIDS (Lambert 1989a) and the fact of a foster care system in major metropolitan areas that is already overtaxed and made more so by the unwillingness of foster families to take black children, fearing they may be AIDS infected (Grossman 1988). A comparative study of racial and cultural variability in survival and support systems of adult women who are diagnosed with AIDS is needed to provide a detailed understanding of the routes through which they manage AIDS, the meanings they attribute to their illness or the illness of a child, and the actions they take as a consequence.

It should be evident by now that, if there were sufficient linkages between sociologists of AIDS, of race and ethnicity, and of the family, important comparative work might be done that explored dimensions and processes of informal caretaking, surely one of the most powerful and subtle aspects of this epidemic. How is it that people (fictive and biological kin) are managing to care for one another in the face of fear, stigma, poverty, fragmented social relations, racism, and heterosexism? It is amazing that there is virtually no examination by sociologists of the nature of caring within the lesbian/gay community, that there are no field or participant observation studies of "mothers of PWAs" or the religious orders who take care of children with AIDS, that no one is systematically looking at how the kinship system of black women is working in dealing with AIDS or at whether or not grandparents' strongly felt rights and responsibilities to grandchildren in Mexican American families has lessened the impact of AIDS in poor and working-class families. Documentation of these patterns is important in showing significant social organization where little is assumed and in demonstrating the strengths and limits of families and communities, thus contributing to policy initiatives focused on the development of local institutional support systems.

Natural neighbors and informal caregivers may be the prime sources of help available to poor people in distress. How has response to AIDS among various groups reflected the 1980s trend to increased medical self-care and increased self-help mutual aid? In what ways has AIDS contributed to the growth of the lay helping system and its integration with professional medical systems and psychosocial services? What are the implications?

A last area for research addresses itself to women and prevention of AIDS. There is as yet little systematic evidence to indicate what interactional or practical difficulties women encounter when they introduce condoms into a sexual scene or talk about changing sexual practice. The age groups most affected by AIDS are precisely those that never had to negotiate male-centered contraception. Young men may have no experience with condoms. Some evidence indicates that women occasionally experience violence by their partners when they try to raise the issue of safer sex and the use of condoms (Richardson 1988). This introduction of a change in sexual terms necessarily reveals the structured nature of gender in sexual relations (Schneider and Gould 1987, p. 125). Much of the prevention material urges women to be even more responsible for sex than they were in the past, locating women as controllers of men's sexuality. Two of the four recent books about AIDS expressly for women base their arguments on the belief that men are not to be trusted in sexual matters (Kaplan 1987; Norwood 1987).

Among the researchable issues that demand systematic, cross-cultural exploration are these: How do women assess their risk given inconsistent reports about heterosexual transmission (Masters, Johnson, and Kolodny 1988; Gould 1988; Leishman 1987)? How and what kinds of sexual partners are chosen by single, heterosexually active women? In what ways is safer sex negotiated when the cultural taboo against sexual talk, especially for heterosexual women, continues to exist (Webster 1984; Laws and Schwartz 1977; Rubin 1976)?

RACIAL/ETHNIC PEOPLES AND COMMUNITIES

The 1980s have been a period of increased racism in the United States. Added to a new visibility of white supremacist groups is the rising racism in educational institutions, professional sports, and the judicial system, from local levels to the Supreme Court. There has been a relatively systematic, though often denied, federal posture of neglect toward African Americans, other people of color, and the poor generally. It is in this environment that talk about AIDS and racial/ethnic peoples must occur. Race framed the epidemiological targeting of an entire nationality, the Haitians, as a "high-risk" group, a political process that requires a social history analysis to sort out and understand, especially because it is likely that the focus on the Haitians diverted attention from U.S. racial/ethnic groups.

It may be that the purported resistance of cultural minority leaders to acknowledging AIDS as a problem has deterred research scholars in this area. Very little has yet to be published by social scientists that systematically explores this resistance. More important, the institutional response to AIDS that has emerged within these communities is, for the most part, undocumented. In New York City, for example, comparative social histories would be appropriate that examined simultaneously the community-based responses of African American, Puerto Rican, and Haitian populations to the threat of AIDS.

What actually were the sources of resistance to dealing with AIDS? How much of the conjecture and commentary by insiders and outsiders alike is accurate? Did homophobia, the stigma of the disease, the fear of ostracism, and increased direct racial assaults impede community leaders (Lee 1989)? Were early twentieth-century racial myths that held blacks responsible for syphilis (Fee 1988; Hammonds 1987) barriers to action? Was fear of deportation a hindrance for Mexican Americans? Were the sources of resistance similar in Latino and black communities? Is it the case that Latino community members were more willing to talk about drugs than sex and African American communities were more willing to talk about sex than drugs?

A second set of questions concerns the mobilization that has occurred in many racial/ethnic communities. A recent survey of over 3,000 U.S. adults indicates clearly that Latinos and blacks are very personally concerned about AIDS, they fear it more than any other disease, and a sizable plurality have made significant changes in their lives. How has this process of change occurred and what do these changes mean? What resources and what institutions have been used by particular communities to respond to HIV? In the mobilization that has occurred, what has been the role of the traditionally active leaders and institutions (like churches) in black and the various Latino communities? Has the impetus for action come from outside, from new groups within the community, or from traditionally silent persons (such as racial/ethnic gay men)? The institutional response of churches is crucial in understanding the cultural minority response to AIDS prevention. In Los Angeles, the Catholic Archdiocese, in reconciling its various contradictory beliefs especially about homosexuality, birth control, and condoms, is making a difference in the kinds of ministerial and educational efforts addressed to Latinos (Horrigan 1988). In other cities, this has not happened. In 1989, black churches in New York City asserted public leadership for the first time.

Class cleavages within each racial/ethnic group suggest a third avenue of research. For example, how does AIDS reveal the management of contradictions within the black community between increased political power, on the one hand, and persistent poverty, on the other? Likewise, given the divergent interests and cultural values of segments within their community, has AIDS divided the various portions of the Mexican American/Chicano community in its response to some of the political, social, and medical dimensions of AIDS.

Inevitably, recognition of both cultural similarities and cultural diversity among Latinos must occur in research endeavors around AIDS. There are sufficient differences among them in terms of income and education level, social organization, citizenship status, political power, and cultural identity to warrant analyzing separately the experiences of Haitians, Puerto Ricans, Cuban Americans, and Chicanos/Mexican Americans, not to mention recent immigrants from Central and South America.

As a number of the earlier discussions indicate, homophobia is posited as a crucial factor in understanding the reactions to AIDS in the lesbian/gay community, among the various racial/ethnic groups, and by heterosexual men. Sociologists need to tackle this heavily psychologized construct of homophobia. Here is a concept whose use is great but whose meaning is vague: the "I know it when I see it" attitude prevails in sociological and other discourse. The term *homophobia* tends to pathologize the social, cultural, and economic structures of power and suggests that the full range of psychological anxieties about homosexuals and homosexuality can be understood in terms of a single cause.

How is homophobia manifested by gender and among different racial/ethnic groups? Systematic investigation into the context and source of homophobia is now warranted in response to increasingly prevalent essays by scholars and activists about homophobia and lesbian baiting in African American (Lorde 1978) and Latino communities (Worth and Rodriguez 1987; Peterson and Marin 1988). How is the fear of homosexuals expressed by critical professionals in an AIDS epidemic (nurses, doctors, politicians)? Why do heterosexual males show consistently higher rates of homophobia than females? How do these feelings or beliefs find expression in violence against lesbians and gay men (Berrill and Burns 1984) and in the resistance of heterosexual males to efforts at education? In addition, further sociological analyses are necessary on the relationship of homophobia to sexual practice, political mobilization, social organization, and kinship and relationships within lesbian/gay communities. And feminist scholars might consider the further theoretical development of the more general and structural notion of heterosexism.

MOBILIZATION OF AFFECTED PEOPLES AND COMMUNITIES

When we talk about mobilization around AIDS, the demand on services, and challenges to entrenched systems, we are exploring the ways in which those who are underrepresented or invisible in government put forward a political agenda in less than ideal ideological and economic conditions (Altman 1987; Shilts 1987), one in which systematic dismantling of the social programs and community action projects of the previous two decades had already occurred. I have little doubt that social movement theory can make a contribution to understanding these processes.

Central to this effort is the need for the systematic examination of the impact of this health crisis on the lesbian/gay movement, the lesbian/gay community, and on individual processes of "coming out." Comparative analyses of the responses of large, urban gay communities (Chicago, New York, Los Angeles) are long overdue; comparative analyses of the variety of, and changes in, small city responses to AIDS by their lesbian/gay organizations and their racial/ethnic communities are increasingly necessary.

As Shaw (1988) documents in her analysis of community organizing efforts, the course of mobilization for women and ethnic minority communities necessarily differs from that of the gay community given aggregate differences in wealth and political power and, hence, in the ability to marshall resources. One of the most challenging, but potentially fruitful, ways to note the differences as well as understand racial dynamics in the AIDS crisis is to study the processes through which the large urban AIDS organizations (AIDS Action Committee—Boston, AIDS Project—Los Angeles, San Francisco AIDS Foundation, Gay Men's Health Crisis—New York)—developed and sustained by resources and volunteers generated primarily by gay men—confront the changing demographics of AIDS patients. What has been the history thus far of competition and accommodation? Have new social movement organizations resulted from resistance of the original groups or from their encouragement and support? And how have contests among groups concerned with AIDS created the basis for structural innovation and new relations in the society?

In most large cities, there has been a proliferation of AIDS organizations as the lack of governmental funds and municipal services placed responsibility for the crisis squarely on the shoulders of the communities most affected. The emergence of a private sector of nonprofit organizations devoted to AIDS, reliant on volunteers from the lesbian/gay community, partially masked the failure of, or virtual lack of, health care delivery. Both structural and ideological analyses of the efforts of these organizations are needed. How do the internal activities of these groups, and the fact that many of their hardest working members may die, affect the strategy and tactics they undertake? Have these groups developed coherent movement cultures that militate against the processes of growth, diversity, and bureaucratization? And, finally, there are organizations composed primarily of people living with AIDS that have entered into a variety of political coalitions locally and nationally. What are the social and policy implications of alliances made, for example, between people with AIDS and disabled persons' associations or conservative groups who object to the Food and Drug Administration as one part of a too-powerful federal government?

POLICY

Sociologists are just beginning to make contributions to the analysis of how social policy around AIDS is being made at the local, state, or federal levels. Who are the interest groups? How do they understand their stakes? What compromises are made? What alliances formed? These are complicated, historically contingent questions, opening up the possibility of collaboration of colleagues in social movements, race and ethnicity, political sociology, and sexuality.

Analyses are needed of the government's response to demands from people with AIDS and how these demands have changed over time as the medical situation alters and as the demographics of new cases change. Conversely, studies also are needed to track the impact of seemingly unrelated policy—such as cuts in California state funding for family planning (Scott 1989) or the abandonment of public services in neighborhoods in New York City—on the lives of HIV-infected people. The state may mobilize resources; it may also initiate repression. How have the various components of governmental and social control apparatuses responded to demand? With regard to AIDS, state apparatuses at various governmental levels organize policies through enforcement of discrimination law, control of education, procedures to detain and punish, and funding.

I will briefly note three policy domains in which systematic investigation is just under way. First, for women, AIDS threatens to legalize and medicalize further the processes of pregnancy and childbirth (Rothman 1987; Zimmerman 1987). Women are in a particularly critical situation in this regard as the implications of some policy proposals force them to confront ethical and rights issues unique to women. The combination of new reproductive surveillance technologies, discussions of fetal rights, and the posing of women's rights against the rights of the fetus are all made manifest in discussions of both AIDS and drug epidemics (Pollitt 1990). Renewed attention is called to women's rights to control sexual practice, women's rights to privacy, and women's rights to be pregnant (Terry 1989; Murphy 1988).

Recent Supreme Court and lower court decisions have a bearing on the kinds of ethical dilemmas and practical choices women will face. Access to abortion and prenatal care are class issues; freedom of choice without economic means to avail oneself of the choice is meaningless. The poor have had the fewest opportunities to exercise control over reproductive activities. The recent incarceration of drug-using pregnant women serves to further exaggerate the problems for select groups of women. The ethical issues raised for individual women have social scientific parallel questions. Among them are: (a)What is the decision-making strategy women use or will use to weigh these often competing rights? (b) How have various communities responded to public messages to curtail sexual activity or forgo childbearing, or to the threat of mandatory abortions for infected pregnant women? and (c) Among organized groups already concerned about issues such as sex education or abortion and family planning, what additional political struggles have emerged and how, if at all, has AIDS changed their political discourse?

Second, services currently available to HIV-infected persons and those with AIDS reflect the complexities of racial, class, and sexual inequities. The AIDS epidemic has revealed these inequalities as well as the already existing gaps in housing and health care. It has brought forward questions about health care and challenges to welfare state policy of a third federal administration and many state and local ones. Where are sociologists when "prominent business executives, concerned about AIDS and over-crowding in hospitals, meet to seek more state aid and even more taxes to pay for services" (Lambert 1989b, p. B1)? AIDS makes problematic the distribution of medical and social services in the United States and suggests comparative analyses of management of AIDS in the United States and other comparable industrialized nations.

Further, health economists have demonstrated that hospitalization is the largest single contributor to costs for AIDS care, and others have shown that the ideal is to treat patients with HIV-related disease on an outpatient, home care, and hospice basis. How have cities and nations responded to these undisputed economic facts? What does it mean to have a federal government put forward plans to fund prevention but not care, especially after its own agency, the Centers for Disease Control, urged medical treatment for all HIV-infected persons? Moreover, how have low-income patients, who cannot buy medical care and have no health insurance, responded to AIDS? This is a question that would have short-term gains but long-term relevance to understanding the situation of the 37 million uninsured people in the United States. In addition, given the increasing numbers of available medicines and alternative healing possi-bilities, a systematic class analysis is needed of asymptomatic persons of all sexes and races to make sense of their conception of, and decisions about, health choices, their illness behaviors in regard to remedial action, the use of sources of help (Mechanic 1986), and their access to AZT and other drugs.

Directly related to the question of service provision are the nationwide controversies regarding placement of community residential facilities for the mentally ill, the homeless, and the retarded. Already there have been outraged reactions to placement of hospices for PWAs and homes for children with AIDS in residential neighborhoods. Systematic analyses of these controversies focusing on variation in geographic locale, population served (gay men, minority persons, children), media coverage, and past history with issues of deinstitutionalization seem likely to reveal the ways in which race and class relations intersect in urban politics.

A third policy domain lies in the area of drug use. How is the gap between the need for treatment facilities for drug users and the level of service being mediated in various locales? For example, in New York City alone, estimates suggest that there is a potential caseload of 250,000 IV drug users, with places for only 43,000. These figures, familiar to those working on social welfare or urban politics, highlight the nature of the emergency and the lack of services even when life-threatening disease is present. With a national government intolerant of drugs, what are the social and economic forces that sustain a lack of drug treatment facilities? How might sociologists account for the fact that the bulk of public policy concerning drugs centers on increased police surveillance of neighborhoods and federal interdiction of drug shipments.

Finally, as Brandt (1985) demonstrated, diseases become social symbols for the anxieties and fears of the cultural milieux in which they emerge. AIDS became public in a political and social terrain in which the issue of changing gender relations and the impact and meaning of a decade's sexual revolution were quite controversial. AIDS, as a medical matter, rapidly became joined, as a structural and social problem, to already heated debate about sexual privacy, reproductive freedom, the viability of relationships that were not heterosexually married and monogamous, and sex education.

Research is needed on the ways in which small segments of the population, right-wing organizations, or fundamentalist religious organizations have affected state and national AIDS policy and public practice around issues such as the introduction and content of sex education and the location and scripts of condom advertisements (Aiken 1987). Ironies of law and practice, such as the continued criminalization of homosexuality in one half the states while safer sex is being taught to gay men, are worthy projects for examination as well. And, certainly, no AIDS-related research agenda is complete without the call for systematic investigation of interactional and institutional dynamics in discrimination against HIV-infected persons.

CONCLUSION

AIDS was, and still is, something that is happening to other people. When the other people are "fags," "hookers," and "junkies," a situation exists in which some do not have to care about others. The majority of people with AIDS are not, given dominant cultural meanings, "innocent victims." That this is true has made AIDS, the medical problem, a formidable sociological challenge. Sociological thinking about research on AIDS and gender, race, and class requires reaching across narrow specializations, caring about IV drug users and gay men in a climate shaped by ideologies of "zero tolerance" and "traditional nuclear families." Sociologists cannot compete with the biomedical establishment that acts as if it owns AIDS. Nevertheless, a consideration of the ways in which AIDS and the relations of race, gender, and class intersect point to important sociological and practical contributions very much needed and as yet to be done.

REFERENCES

Adam, Barry. 1978. *The Survival of Domination: Inferiorization and Everyday Life.* New York: Elsevier-North Holland.

"AIDS Testing Without Consent Reported." 1988. *New York Times,* January 9, p. A7.

Aiken, Jane Harris. 1987. "Education as Prevention." Pp. 90-105 in *AIDS and the Law,* edited by H. Dalton, S. Burris, and the Yale AIDS Law Project. New Haven, CT: Yale University Press.

Albert, Edward. 1986. "Illness and Deviance: The Response of the Press to AIDS." Pp. 163-78 in *The Social Dimensions of AIDS,* edited by D. Feldman and T. M. Johnson. New York: Praeger.

Altman, Dennis. 1987. *AIDS in the Mind of America.* New York: Anchor.

Andrade, Sally. 1982. "Social Science Stereotypes of the Mexican-American Woman: Policy Implications for Research." *Hispanic Journal of Behavior Science* 4:223-44.

Bell, Alan P. and Martin S. Weinberg. 1978. *Homosexualities: A Study of Diversity Among Men and Women.* New York: Simon & Schuster.

Berk, Richard A. 1987. "Anticipating the Social Consequences of AIDS: A Position Paper." *American Sociologist* 18:3-33.

Bernard, Jesse. 1981. "The Good Provider: Its Rise and Fall." *American Psychologist* 36:1-12.

Berrill, Kevin and J. Burns. 1984. "NGTF Violence Survey Indicates Anti-Gay/Lesbian Violence Widespread." *National Gay Task Force Newsletter* 11:1.

Bowser, Benjamin. 1988. "Crack and AIDS: An Ethnographic Impression." *Multicultural Inquiry and Research on AIDS Quarterly Newsletter* 2:1-2.

Brandt, Alan. 1985. *No Magic Bullet: A Social History of Venereal Disease in the United States Since 1880.* New York: Oxford University Press.

Callen, Michael. 1988. "I Will Survive." *Village Voice,* May 3, p. 31.

Collins, Patricia Hill. 1986. "Learning From the Outsider Within: The Social Significance of Black Feminist Thought." *Social Problems* 33:S14-S32.

Conrad, Peter. 1989. "The Social Reaction to AIDS as a Social Problem: Notes for Discussion." Paper presented at the American Sociological Association Workshop on researching AIDS. Miami, May.

Dawson, D. A. and O. T. Thornberry. 1988. "AIDS Knowledge and Attitudes for Hispanics." National Center for Health Statistics, Publication No. PHS 88-1250. Washington, DC: Government Printing Office.

Des Jarlais, Don, C. Casriel, and Samuel R. Friedman. 1988. "The New Death Among IV Drug Users." Pp. 135-50 in *AIDS: Principles, Practices, and Politics,* edited by I. Corless and M. Pittman-Lindeman. Washington, DC: Hemisphere.

Des Jarlais, Don and Samuel R. Friedman. 1988. "The Psychology of Preventing AIDS Among IV Drug Users: A Social Learning Conceptualization." *American Psychologist* 43:865-70.

Des Jarlais, Don, Samuel R. Friedman, and David Strug. 1986. "AIDS and Needle Sharing Within the IV-Drug Subculture." Pp. 111-25 in *Social Dimensions of AIDS,* edited by D. A. Feldman and T. A. Johnson. New York: Praeger.

DiClemente, Ralph, Cherrie Boyer, and Edward S. Morales. 1988. "Minorities and AIDS: Knowledge, Attitudes, and Misconceptions Among Black and Latino Adolescents." *American Journal of Public Health* 78:55-57.

Epstein, Stephen. 1987. "Gay Politics, Ethnic Identity: The Limits of Social Constructionism." *Socialist Review* 17:9-54.

Ergas, Yasmine. 1987. "The Social Consequences of the AIDS Epidemic." *Social Science Research Council* 41(December):33-39.

Fee, Elizabeth. 1988. "Sin vs. Science: Venereal Disease in 20th Century Baltimore." Pp. 121-46 in *AIDS: The Burdens of History,* edited by E. Fee and D. Fox. Berkeley: University of California Press.

Fineberg, Harvey. 1988. "Education to Prevent AIDS: Prospects and Obstacles." *Science* 239:592-96.

Foster, Jim. 1988. "Impact of the AIDS Epidemic on the Gay Political Agenda." Pp. 209-19 in *AIDS: Principles, Practices and Politics,* edited by I. Corless and M. Pittman-Lindeman. Washington, DC: Hemisphere.

Foster, Zelda. 1988. "The Treatment of People with AIDS: Psychosocial Considerations." Pp. 33-45 in *AIDS: Principles, Practices and Politics,* edited by I. Corless and M. Pittman-Lindeman. Washington, DC: Hemisphere.

Friedman, Samuel R., Don C. Des Jarlais, Jo L. Sotheran, Jonathan Garber, Henry Cohen, and Donald Smith. 1987. "AIDS and Self-Organization Among Intravenous Drug Users." *International Journal of the Addictions* 22:201-19.

Gagnon, John. 1989. "Notes for Miami ASA Meeting." Paper presented at the American Sociological Association Workshop on researching AIDS." Miami, May.

Gould, Robert E. 1988. "Reassuring News About AIDS: A Doctor Tells Why You May Not Be at Risk." *Cosmopolitan*, January.

Grossman, Moses. 1988. "Children with AIDS." Pp. 167-73 in *AIDS: Principles, Practices and Politics*, edited by I. Corless and M. Pittman-Lindeman. Washington, DC: Hemisphere.

Hammonds, Evelynn. 1987. "Race, Sex, AIDS: The Construction of 'Other.'" *Radical America* 20:28-36.

Horrigan, Alice. 1988. "AIDS and the Catholic Church." Pp. 83-113 in *The Social Impact of AIDS in the U.S.*, edited by R. A. Berk. Cambridge, MA: Abt.

Interrante, Joseph. 1987. "To Have Without Holding: Memories of Life With a Person With AIDS." *Radical America* 20:55-62.

Johnson, Paula, Doralba Munoz, and Jose Pares. 1988. "Multicultural Concerns and AIDS Action: Creating an Alternative." *Radical America* 21:24-33.

Kaplan, Helen Singer. 1987. *The Real Truth About Women and AIDS: How to Eliminate Risks Without Giving Up Love and Sex*. New York: Simon & Schuster.

Kaplan, Howard, ed. 1983. *Psychosocial Stress: Trends in Theory and Research*. New York: Academic Press.

Kayal, Philip M. 1989. "Healing Maladaptive Sexual Behavior." Paper presented at the meetings of the Society for the Study of Social Problems. New York, August.

Lambert, Bruce. 1989a. "AIDS Legacy: A Growing Generation of Orphans." *New York Times*, July 17, p. A1.

———. 1989b "U.S. Urging Vast Effort to Treat Million People Infected with AIDS Virus." *New York Times*, July 8, p. 25.

Laws, Judith and Pepper Schwartz. 1977. *Sexual Scripts: The Social Construction of Female Sexuality*. Hinsdale, IL: Dryden.

Lee, Felicia. 1989. "Black Doctors Urge Study of Factors in Risk of AIDS." *New York Times*, July 21, p. B7.

Leishman, Katie. 1987. "Heterosexuals and AIDS: The Second Stage of the Epidemic." *Atlantic Monthly*, February, pp. 39-58.

Lorde, Audre. 1984. *Sister/Outsider*. New York: Crossing Press.

Luker, Kristin. 1975. *Taking Chances: Abortion and the Decision Not to Contracept*. Berkeley: University of California Press.

Macks, Judith and Dan Turner. 1986. "Mental Health Issues of Persons with AIDS." Pp. 111-24 in *What to Do About AIDS: Physicians and Mental Health Professionals Discuss the Issues*, edited by L. McKusick. Berkeley: University of California Press.

Mandel, Jeffrey S. 1986. "Psychosocial Challenges of AIDS and ARC: Clinical and Research Observations." Pp. 75-86 in *What to Do About AIDS: Physicians and Mental Health Professionals Discuss the Issues*, edited by L. McKusick. Berkeley: University of California Press.

Magura, S., J. I. Grossman, and D. S. Lipton. 1989. "Determinants of Needle Sharing Among Intravenous Drug Users." *American Journal of Public Health* 79:459-62.

Masters, William H., Virginia E. Johnson, and R. C. Kolodny. 1988. *Crisis: Heterosexual Behavior in the Age of AIDS*. New York: Grove.

McKusick, Leon, W. Horstman, and T. J. Coates. 1986. "AIDS and Sexual Behavior Reported by Gay Men in San Francisco." *American Journal of Public Health* 75:493-96.

Mechanic, David. 1986. "Illness Behavior: An Overview." Pp. 101-8 in *Illness Behavior: A Multidisciplinary Model*, edited by S. McHugh and T. M. Vallis. New York: Plenum.

Moore, Joan and Mary Devitt. 1989. "The Paradox of Deviance in Addicted Mexican American Mothers." *Gender & Society* 3:53-70.

Murphy, Julien S. 1988. "Women With AIDS: Sexual Ethics in an Epidemic." Pp. 65-79 in *AIDS: Principles, Practices, and Politics*, edited by I. Corless and M. Pittman-Lindeman. Washington, DC: Hemisphere.

National Academy of Sciences. 1986. *Mobilizing Against AIDS*. Cambridge, MA: Harvard University Press.

Norwood, Chris. 1987. *Advice for Life: A Woman's Guide to AIDS Risks and Prevention*. New York: Pantheon.

O'Connell, M. 1980. "Comparative Estimates of Teenage Illegitimacy in the United States, 1940-44 to 1970-74." *Demography*, 17:13-24.

O'Neill, Catherine. 1987. "Intravenous Drug Users." Pp. 253-80 in *AIDS and the Law*, edited by H. Dalston, S. Burris, and the Yale AIDS Law Project. New Haven, CT: Yale University Press.

Peterson, John L. and Gerardo Marin. 1988. "Issues in the Prevention of AIDS Among Black and Hispanic Men." *American Psychologist* 43:871-77.

Pollitt, Katha. 1990. " 'Fetal Rights': A New Assault on Feminism." *The Nation*, March 26, pp. 409-18.

"Pregnant Women to Get AIDS Drug in Test." 1989. *New York Times*, July 11, p. C.2.

Richardson, Diane. 1988. *Women and AIDS*. New York: Methuen.

Robins, Lee. 1980. "The Natural History of Drug Abuse." In *Theories of Drug Abuse* (National Institute of Drug Abuse). Washington, DC: Government Printing Office.

Rosen, Don. 1986. "LA Gay Men Reduce Unsafe Sex Practices, Survey Finds." *Los Angeles Times*, March 21, p. 1.

Rosenbaum, Marsha. 1981. *Women on Heroin*. New Brunswick, NJ: Rutgers University Press.

Rothman, Barbara Katz. 1987. "Reproduction." Pp. 154-89 in *Analyzing Gender*, edited by B. Hess and M. M. Ferree. Newbury Park, CA: Sage.

Rubin, Lillian. 1976. *Worlds of Pain: Life in the Working-Class Family*. New York: Stein and Day.

Sabogal, R., G. Marin, R. Otero-Sabogal, B. V. Marin, and E. J. Perez-Stable. 1987. "Hispanic Familism and Acculturation: What Changes and What Doesn't." *Hispanic Journal of Behavioral Sciences* 9:397-412.

Schneider, Beth E. 1988. "Gender, Sexuality and AIDS: Social Responses and Consequences." Pp. 15-36 in *The Social Impact of AIDS in the U.S.*, edited by R. A. Berk. Cambridge, MA: Abt.

Schneider, Beth E. and Meredith Gould. 1987. "Female Sexuality: Looking Back Into the Future." Pp. 120-53 in *Analyzing Gender*, edited by B. Hess and M. M. Ferree. Newbury Park, CA: Sage.

Scott, Janny. 1989. "Family Clinic Funding Cutbacks Hit Poor Hardest, Officials Say." *Los Angeles Times*, July 28, p. 3.

Selik, R. M., K. G. Castro, and M. Peppaioanov. 1988. "Racial/Ethnic Differences in the Risk of AIDS in the United States." *American Journal of Public Health* 78:1539-45.

Shaw, Nancy Stoller. 1988. "Preventing AIDS Among Women: The Role of Community Organizing." *Socialist Review* 18:76-92.

Shaw, Nancy Stoller and Lyn Paleo. 1986. "Women and AIDS." Pp. 142-54 in *What to Do About AIDS: Physicians and Mental Health Professionals Discuss the Issues*, edited by L. McKusick. Berkeley: University of California Press.

Shilts, Randy. 1987. *And the Band Played On: Politics, People and the AIDS Epidemic.* New York: St. Martin's.

Sontag, Susan. 1988. *AIDS and Its Metaphors.* New York: Farrar, Straus and Giroux.

Terry, Jennifer. 1989. "The Body Invaded: Medical Surveillance of Women as Reproducers." *Socialist Review* 3:13-43.

Thompson, K. 1980. "A Comparison of Black and White Adolescents Beliefs About Having Children." *Journal of Marriage and the Family* 42:133-40.

Treichler, Paula A. 1988. "AIDS, Homophobia, and Biomedical Discourse: An Epidemic of Signification." Pp. 31-70 in *AIDS: Cultural Analysis, Cultural Activism,* edited by D. Crimp. Cambridge: MIT Press.

Webster, Paula. 1984. "The Forbidden: Eroticism and Taboo." Pp. 385-98 in *Pleasure and Danger: Exploring Female Sexuality,* edited by C. Vance. Boston: Routledge & Kegan Paul.

Williams, L. S. 1986. "AIDS Risk Reduction: A Community Health Education Intervention for Minority High-Risk Group Members." *Health Education Quarterly* 13:407-21.

Worth, Dooley and Ruth Rodriguez. 1987. "Latina Women and AIDS." *Radical America* 20:63-67.

Zelnick, M. and J. Kanter. 1980. "Sexual Activity, Contraceptive Use and Pregnancy Among Metropolitan-Area Teenagers: 1971-1979." *Family Planning Perspectives* 12:230-37.

Zimmerman, Mary K. 1987. "The Women's Health Movement: A Critique of Medical Enterprise and the Position of Women." Pp. 442-72 in *Analyzing Gender,* edited by B. Hess and M. M. Ferree. Newbury Park, CA: Sage.

Zimmerman, Rick S. 1989. "Sociology's Potential Contributions Toward Research on Sexual Behavior and the Prevention of HIV-Related Disease." Paper presented at the American Sociological Association Workshop on researching AIDS. Miami, May.

Part II
The Social Context
of Risky Behavior

3

Unprotected Sex:
Understanding Gay Men's Participation

Martin P. Levine
Karolynn Siegel

In the absence of a curative treatment or vaccination, behavioral change remains the most effective means for curtailing the spread of the human immunodeficiency virus (HIV) epidemic (Coates 1990). Individuals must be persuaded to refrain from practices associated with the transmission of infection (Institute of Medicine 1988), which, in the case of gay men, primarily include unprotected anal and oral intercourse (Turner, Miller, and Moses 1989). Accordingly, HIV prevention efforts aimed at the gay community have encouraged the use of condoms during insertive and receptive anal and oral sex and have presented protected intercourse as a socially acceptable and responsible action (Siegel, Grodsky, and Herman 1986; Connell et al. 1989).

Prevention campaigns have succeeded in fostering some normative, attitudinal, and behavioral change with respect to protected sex among gay men living in epicenters of HIV infection (Turner et al. 1989). Prior to AIDS, cultural rules within these gay communities proscribed condom usage during homosexual relations (Williams 1979). Gay men perceived condoms as chiefly a contraceptive device and thus irrelevant to same-sex

AUTHORS' NOTE: Ordering of the authors' names is alphabetical. Both authors have made an equal contribution to this chapter. This work was supported by a grant from the National Institute of Mental Health (MH42275). We wish to acknowledge the assistance of Dr. Beatrice Krauss, Shona Brogden, and Dr. Stephen O. Murray.

contacts. Moreover, the easy availability of curative treatments for most venereal diseases prompted gay men to eschew condoms as a prophylaxis against these illnesses (Judson 1977). In this sense, gay men considered the health risks of unprotected intercourse as acceptable when weighed against the perceived sexual and psychological benefits. Hence, prophylaxis was rarely considered or used during homosexual acts (Martin 1987; Ross 1988a).

However, the threat of HIV disease has transformed norms and attitudes toward protected anal sex within gay communities located in areas that are the foci of the epidemic (Stall, Coates, and Hoff 1988; Becker and Joseph 1988). Available evidence suggests that gay men dwelling in these communities now regard unprotected anal intercourse as an extremely efficient means of transmitting HIV and condom use as a normative, necessary, and effective means of preventing infection during anal sex (Turner et al. 1989). For example, in 1987 Communication Technologies researchers asked a random probability sample of self-identified gay and bisexual men living in San Francisco to rate the risk of HIV transmission during unprotected anal sex on a 10-point scale on which 10 indicated that this practice was very associated with the risk of transmission and 1 indicated it was not associated with transmission. The mean reported risk score was 9.8. In addition, the investigators questioned the sample about the extent to which they agreed with the following two statements: (a) "The only way I will have anal sex is with a condom." (b)"Most of my friends believe that I should only have anal intercourse with a condom." Again, a 10-point scale was used on which 10 represented complete agreement. The mean acceptance score for the first statement was 8.2; for the second it was 8.8.

Significant behavioral modifications of anal sexual practices have paralleled these normative and attitudinal shifts (Stall et al. 1988; Becker and Joseph 1988). Survey data from gay men residing in cities with high rates of HIV infection indicate striking increases in the frequency of protected anal intercourse (Martin 1987; McKusick, Wiley et al. 1985; McKusick, Hortsman, and Coates 1985; Siegel, Bauman, Christ, and Krown 1988a; Stall, McKusick, Wiley, Coates, and Ostrow 1986; Communication Technologies 1987). For example, using longitudinal data from a community-based convenience sample of self-identified gay men living in New York City, Martin, Dean, Gracia, and Hall (1989) found that the percentage of men reporting always using condoms during receptive anal sex increased from 2% in 1981 to 62% in 1987. Similarly, the

percentage indicating always using condoms during insertive anal intercourse rose from 2% in 1981 to 58% in 1987.

Despite these substantial changes, these same surveys also record the
persistence of participation in unprotected anal sex among a significant
percentage of men in epicenter gay communities (Stall et al. 1988; Becker
and Joseph 1988). For example, Communication Technologies (1987)
researchers found that almost one third (31%) of their sample had practiced unprotected anal intercourse with a primary partner during the past
6 months and that 6% of the sample behaved similarly with a secondary
partner during the same time period. Other studies indicate occasional
relapses into unprotected anal sex among a substantial proportion of men
studied (Siegel, Mesagno, Chen, and Christ 1988b; Stall et al. 1986).

Additional data from these surveys suggest minimal changes in norms
or attitudes toward protected oral sex (Turner et al. 1989). Typically, gay
male residents of areas that are at the center of the epidemic perceive oral
sex without ejaculation as an unlikely means of HIV transmission and,
hence, reject protection during this act (Martin et al. 1989). For example,
Communication Technologies (1987) researchers also asked their sample
to rank the risk of HIV transmission during oral sex without semen
exchange (again using a 10-point scale on which 10 indicated the practice
was very associated with transmission and 1 indicated the practice was
not related to transmission). The scores signified that the men regarded
this act as about as risky as protected anal intercourse. The mean reported
risk score for oral sex without ejaculation was 3.7; it was 3.5 for protected
anal intercourse. It is not surprising that unprotected oral sex, albeit
usually without ejaculation or semen ingestion, remains prevalent in
epicenter communities. In fact, Martin et al. (1989) found that, as of 1987,
approximately 85% of their sample had engaged in either unprotected
insertive or receptive oral sex at least once during the past year.

The reasons for the persistence of unprotected intercourse among gay
men living in epicenter communities remain poorly understood. Unfortu-
nately, studies of behavioral change within these locales commonly only
ask questions about the magnitude and correlates of protected inter-
course and rarely directly examine motives for unprotected sex (Coates,
Stall, Catania, and Kegeles 1988; Siegel, Bauman et al. 1988; Siegel,
Mesagno et al. 1988; Martin 1987; Martin et al. 1989; McKusick,
Wiley et al. 1985; McKusick, Hortsman et al. 1985; Stall et al. 1986;
Ross 1988a, 1988b, 1988c; Valdiserri et al. 1987; Valdiserri et al. 1988).
Only one survey tapped gay men's reasons for engaging in unprotected

anal intercourse. In this study (Communication Technologies 1987), researchers found that partner status, condom unavailability, coitus interruptus, condom acceptability, and partner seronegativity were the most frequently offered reasons for unprotected anal sex. More than half (54%) of the sample reported that they eschewed protection because they only had anal sex with primary partners; one quarter (25%) indicated that they did not use protection because condoms were not available; about one fifth (18%) stated that they avoided protection because they withdrew before ejaculation; a similar proportion (18%) reported that they shunned protection because they did not like condoms; and approximately one tenth (13%) indicated that they eschewed protection because both they and their partners were seronegative. To date, then, not much is known about why most gay men perceive oral sex as an inefficient means of transmitting HIV or about why some gay men continue to practice a behavior (unprotected anal sex) that they define as risky.

This chapter expands our understanding of the motives of gay male residents of HIV epicenters for engaging in unprotected intercourse. In what follows, we discuss the research methods used to collect our data on gay men's explanations for this behavior, report the reasons for unprotected intercourse cited by our respondents, and comment upon how the major social constructions of the risk of HIV infection during intercourse and culturally available motives for improper sexual conduct are reflected in our respondents' comments.

Following Scott and Lyman (1968), we conceptualized the men's reports as "accounts" and typologized them as either "justifications" or "excuses." Accounts are culturally determined narrative statements offered to explain untoward or problematic behavior. Justifications assume responsibility for committing the act but deny that it was unseemly or questionable behavior. Excuses admit that the act is improper or inappropriate but dispute culpability for committing it through either scapegoating or appealing to reasons such as accidents, defeasibility, or biological drives.

METHOD

The data presented below are from a qualitative study of sexual decision making among gay men in the context of the AIDS epidemic. The study was undertaken in response to a recognition that, although self-identified gay men have participated in several survey studies concerning the extent to which the AIDS epidemic fostered changes in their sexual lives, there has been a notable lack of research on the meaning of AIDS as it is pragmatically experienced and cognitively structured by the men themselves. The study was designed to address this problem using a primarily qualitative methodology that included participant observation, the use of a brief self-administered questionnaire, and primary reliance on unstructured but focused individual interviews (Merton, Fiske, and Kendall 1956).

Respondents for the study were recruited through flyers distributed and posted at a variety of gay service, political, and social organizations (including the large Lesbian and Gay Community Center, which serves the organized gay community in New York). In addition, recruiting announcements were run as advertisements in gay newspapers and as public service announcements on gay cable television, announced at various gay organizational meetings, published in a range of gay newsletters, and distributed through a constantly growing recruitment network.

To participate, respondents had to be between 18 and 65 years of age, live in greater New York metropolitan area, not have used intravenous drugs in the past 6 months, and not have been diagnosed with AIDS. We excluded intravenous drug users because the study aimed at understanding behavioral change among individuals for whom sexual practices constituted the principal risk behavior. Men with AIDS were not included because we felt that their physical and mental symptomatology might be more significant explanatory factors for their sexual behavior than the kinds of interpersonal, social, and cultural factors we were trying to elucidate.

All interviews were conducted as relatively unstructured open-ended discussions led by the project interviewer. Interview sessions began with a 9-minute videotape produced by the study team as a projective stimulus for discussion. The video contained five vignettes in which actors portrayed gay men articulating their diverse views about safer sex and AIDS. The vignettes included men who had adopted safer sex practices and expressed differing feelings about their choice as well as men who justified continuing to engage in risky sex. By presenting varying views about safer sex, the video was designed to give respondents permission to express themselves candidly (e.g., to acknowledge disagreement with safer sex recommendations or involvement in unsafe sexual practices). Interviews were audiotaped and transcribed verbatim for analysis.

The findings presented here were derived from the focused interviews with a subset of 124 men, out of a total of 150 respondents, who reported having engaged in unprotected anal or oral intercourse (with and without ejaculation) during the preceding 6 months. Of these, 40% were untested, 32% were seropositive, and 29% were seronegative for HIV antibodies. Of the respondents, 110 were white, 6 were Hispanic, 3 were black, and the remaining 5 were from diverse racial and ethnic groups. The mean age of this subsample of respondents was 34, and 78% of the subsample was under 40 years of age. The men were well educated: 94% had completed some undergraduate education, and 71% had completed college or attended graduate school. All interviews were conducted between May 1988 and January 1990.

The data reported below were usually offered in reply to a general query by the interviewer asking respondents to discuss what led to their participation in reported incidents of unprotected sex. The interviewer also directly questioned the men about the context in which these encounters occurred. Because the interviews were unstructured, there were no standardized probes as a follow-up to their responses. That is, the interviewer did not systematically probe to explore the possible importance of factors other than those reported by the men. In this way, we believe that we captured the respondents' subjective perceptions and definition of the situation and gained insight into what factors were personally most salient to them in arriving at their decision to participate in unprotected sex. For the purpose of exposition, we segregated the reasons offered by the men in their accounts of this decision. In reality, their accounts typically contained several interrelated reasons.

ACCOUNTS

The men participating in our study typically regarded unprotected intercourse as improper or problematic behavior and, therefore, readily offered accounts for their actions, which took the form of either justifications or excuses. The men citing justifications intentionally and routinely engaged in unprotected sex. Although these men accepted responsibility for their conduct, they disputed the notion that the behavior risked transmitting HIV. They either openly doubted the validity of a practice's classification as risky (this was limited primarily to unprotected oral sex) or believed they could eliminate, or at least minimize, the risk of HIV transmission during unprotected intercourse through strategies that prevented the transmission of infected body fluids into the bloodstream.

Conversely, the men offering excuses inadvertently and irregularly engaged in unprotected sex. Typically these men perceived participation in unprotected intercourse as risky and, therefore, usually used protection during anal or oral sex. They regarded instances of unprotected sex as an unintended relapse from their normal pattern of protection, which emerged from either "extenuating circumstances" or "external forces" beyond their control.

Justifications

The justifications cited by our respondents generally reflected their perceptions of how HIV was transmitted during intercourse. Typically the men believed that the transmission of HIV required the passage of infected body fluids (blood, semen, or preseminal fluids) directly into the bloodstream through lacerations on the penis or the interior lining of mouth or anus. Our respondents specified that three conditions were required for HIV transmission. First, they believed that either one or both of the partners had to be infected with HIV. Second, they felt that the infected partner had to deposit sufficient quantities of an infected body fluid into the mouth or anus of the uninfected partner. Third, they believed that the infected body fluid had to directly enter the uninfected partner's bloodstream through tears on the skin or lining of the penis, anus, or mouth.

The men offering justifications typically felt that their sexual behavior was not risky because one or more of the conditions required for the transmission of HIV was not present. We have grouped their comments into four categories of reasons: (a) no signs of infectivity, (b) no transmission of either semen and/or preseminal fluids, (c) no lacerations, and (d) the belief that saliva, gastric juices, and urethral acids either inhibit or kill the virus.

No signs of infectivity. Many respondents defended acts of unprotected intercourse on the grounds that both they and/or their partners were known or assumed to be uninfected. Typically these men saw no risk of HIV transmission during unprotected sex between uninfected partners. They regarded unprotected intercourse between an infected and uninfected partner similarly, as long as the uninfected partner took the insertive role or precautions were taken to ensure that infected body fluids did not enter the bloodstream of the uninfected partner.

The men offering this explanation based their presumption of their own or their partners' uninfected status on a variety of medical and social criteria. These men reasoned that either they or their partners were uninfected because there was either medical proof of seronegativity or social indicators of a low-risk status.

Medical evidence of seronegativity. Some men perceived normal T-cell counts and negative HIV antibody test results as medical evidence of their virus-free status. Several, for example, stated that they had unprotected sex with current lovers because they had both tested seronegative for HIV antibodies. One 33-year-old technical writer reported having unprotected oral-genital contact with his lover because "he [the lover] knew he was negative and I knew I was negative, and ah so it seemed that we, neither of us, . . . was at risk." Others mentioned seronegativity as a reason for ceasing protected sex with lovers. For example, a 24-year-old customer service representative who had tested negative told us that he and his lover "stopped using condoms" after they both tested negative. A few men justified having unprotected receptive oral intercourse on the grounds that their partners were seronegative. One man, who was 30 and had tested positive, stated that he fellated his last two lovers without condoms because his lovers were both "negative, and my doctor said that [he did not] see what the risk is." The men typically believed that the insertive partner in oral intercourse was not at risk if there were no tears or cuts on the penis.

Nearly all the men citing seronegativity as a reason for engaging in unprotected sex accepted the validity of their test result. The possibility of a false negative result was almost never mentioned, even by men who were surprised at testing negative or who had had risky sex shortly before taking the test and thus might have not yet seroconverted.

Social evidence of a low-risk status. Other men construed sexual history and geographic locale as social markers of a low-risk status. Some of these men assumed that either they or their partners were not infected because prior to or throughout the epidemic they had been monogamous, relatively sexually inactive, or rarely took the receptive role during anal intercourse, which minimized their chance of exposure to HIV. For example, a 30-year-old waiter who had tested negative told us that he repeatedly had unprotected sex with his former lover because "I thought he was only seeing me . . . and I'm into one man relationships . . . and therefore the possibility of either of us having the virus were slight." An unemployed 24-year-old, who was untested, felt that "fucking" his steady partner was safe because the partner had "been with only one person for five years [and] there's no way [he] could have it." One seronegative 32-year-old Hispanic respondent had a number of episodes of unprotected anal sex with a priest. He explained his behavior by saying that, although he knew he couldn't be "100 percent certain" that the priest was uninfected, he was confident that the priest's life-style had greatly restricted his opportunity for encounters with many different partners and thus limited the probability of his having become infected.

Typical of those who believed that men who either avoided or rarely engaged in receptive anal sex were most likely to be uninfected was an untested college student in his early twenties. He justified regularly fellating his lover without condoms on the grounds that his lover had never been the receptive partner during anal sex, which he presumed meant that his lover was uninfected. He commented:

> I mean I would say that he's at zero risk. He's at virtually none. He ah, he's ten years older than me. He'll be 32 at the end of the month. But he was a virgin until six months before I met him. . . . And he had only had very safe sex with a couple of people before I met him. All of whom I know. Save one, one whom I haven't met. But I know who he is. And ah, he'd only been very very safe. So I don't worry about him at all.

Other respondents assumed that their partners were uninfected because they came from locales with a low prevalence of AIDS cases, and, therefore, probably a low incidence of HIV infection, which greatly diminished their chance of becoming exposed to the virus. These men believed that unprotected intercourse with partners from low-prevalence areas (e.g., Michigan, Canada) who had either recently moved to New York or were just visiting the city was not risky. For example, a 38-year-old Hispanic counselor who was untested explained that he did not use condoms with men who were "imports," that is, partners from countries that he thought had few AIDS cases, because their chances of being infected were minimal. Similarly, men traveling to low-incidence areas either abroad or within the United States felt that they could have unprotected intercourse during these excursions with little fear of becoming infected.

No transmission of either semen and/or preseminal fluids. Some men justified engaging in unprotected receptive intercourse on the grounds that there was no transmission of either ejaculate and/or preejaculatory fluids. There were two subgroups among these respondents. The first consisted of those who defended this practice on the basis of not receiving semen. Almost all of these men regarded ejaculate as transmitting HIV. Accordingly, they felt that they could minimize the danger of infection during receptive sex by avoiding semen. For example, the college student cited above commented on the risk associated with unprotected receptive oral intercourse with his lover:

> We'll give each other blow jobs but won't cum in each other's mouths. Ah, we never ejaculate in each other's mouths. And I consider that pretty safe as well.

Most of these men also regarded preejaculatory fluids as an ineffective transmitter of HIV. Typically they felt that preseminal fluids did not harbor or contain sufficient amounts of the virus to cause infection. Consequently, they believed the fluids posed little risk of transmission of infection to the receptive partner. For example, a 41-year-old accountant who had not been tested justified unprotected receptive anal sex with his lover on the grounds that his lover "didn't cum in me [and] precum isn't a risk factor." Another man, a 35-year-old actor who had not taken the HIV antibody test, doubted that there was enough preejaculatory fluid to transmit the virus during receptive oral intercourse. He based his belief on a conversation with a registered nurse at a community-based health clinic for gay men, who showed him a takeout Chinese food carton and said, "That's how much preejaculation would have to be in your mouth for you to swallow to get AIDS."

The second group defended unprotected receptive oral sex on the basis of not ingesting semen or preseminal fluids. Unlike the first group, these men believed that both ejaculate and preejaculatory fluids carried the virus. Hence, they felt they could minimize the risk of transmission during receptive fellatio by not allowing these body fluids to enter the mouth.

These men described two procedures for avoiding the ingestion of these fluids during oral intercourse. In the first, the receptive partner stimulated the scrotum and the shaft of the penis with his tongue and mouth but did not take the glans (head) of the penis into the mouth and, therefore, avoided ingesting any fluids. A 29-year-old seronegative college student said that he practiced this technique by stimulating "around—but not the head; but sort of around, you know, balls and everything."

In the second procedure, the receptive partner inserted the penile glans and shaft into his mouth only when semen and preseminal fluids were not present. The accountant referred to above, who had sexual relations with a male prostitute while his lover of 19 years was dying from AIDS, believed that the absence of these fluids reduced the risk of unprotected receptive fellatio:

> He [the prostitute] knows by now what I want. Ah, the second time I was with him, I put his cock into my mouth, and I have ever since. He has no precum. . . . You know I've tried putting a condom on him. But he has no precum and I say, "Well, it's basically safe" and he doesn't cum. He doesn't have an orgasm with me. Which again is fine. You know what I'm saying? All I want is to get off, and have some enjoyment that's safe and "bye."

Similarly, a 33-year-old journalist who did not yet know the results of his HIV antibody test told us that he regarded receptive fellatio as safe when his partners were "dry." He said:

> If I see that the person tends to be ah, to have precum, I don't go down on him. If I see that the person tends to be dry and the person is attractive and I feel like it, then I would maybe go as far as taking it in my mouth.

No lacerations. Many men justified engaging in unprotected sex on the grounds that there were no tears, sores, or cuts on the skin or lining of the penis, anus, or mouth. Almost all these men believed that HIV-infected body fluids entered the bloodstream during intercourse through either anal, oral, or genital lacerations. Moreover, they felt that these tears commonly occurred during receptive anal sex, largely because of the friction associated with the thrusting of the penis and the fragility of the interior walls of the anus. Hence, they believed that receptive anal intercourse was quite risky.

Nevertheless, most of these respondents openly doubted the risk classification of insertive anal and receptive oral intercourse. Usually these men felt that lacerations were generally absent during these practices, which prevented infected body fluids from entering the bloodstream. They believed that tears rarely occurred during insertive anal sex because the sphincter muscles of the receptive partner were usually relaxed and thus penetration did not lacerate either the interior of the anus or the skin of the penis. The journalist, quoted above, who did not know the results of his HIV antibody test, told us:

> I must say that I feel there is virtually no danger in penetrating unless there is a great deal of pain and laceration and whatever else. Otherwise I feel that if everything is relaxed then there is no great danger.

Later in the interview he continued:

> Penetrating another guy without a condom? I tend to believe that it's not risky. Again, unless you are putting a great deal of effort in penetration, then there's lesions and all that. When it just comes real easy and natural, when it's smooth, then I feel that it's OK.

These men also discounted the likelihood of wounds during receptive oral sex on the grounds that most men rarely had bleeding gums or sores in their mouths. A 44-year-old hair stylist who tested positive said that "oral sex is not, unless you have sores or lesions in your mouth, as difficult or as dangerous as everybody thinks." The actor, referred to above, who was counseled by the nurse at the community-based health clinic, felt similarly and said:

> I think that oral sex is safer [than anal sex]. I do think that if you have bleeding gums or sores in your mouth or herpes sores on your mouth, you run a great risk.

He again based his belief on what the nurse told him, which was this:

> Having someone perform oral sex on you is low risk. The only way that it could be risky to you is if someone was performing on you if they have severe cuts all the way in the back of their mouth, periodontal problems.

A handful of respondents felt that the absence of lacerations precluded risk even during receptive oral sex with ejaculation. Typical of those who believed this was a 32-year-old, HIV-antibody positive, writer, who commented:

> I will have oral sex. The subject of ejaculation has not come up lately but I honestly think that, theoretically, to me, that it is OK. I'm assuming that one did not floss twenty minutes ago [causing bleeding gums].

Saliva, gastric juices, and urethral acids either inhibit or kill the virus. Many men justified engaging in unprotected intercourse on the grounds that saliva, gastric juices, and urethral acids either destroyed or inhibited the infectivity of HIV. There were two subgroups among these respondents. The first consisted of those who defended the ingestion of either ejaculate or preejaculatory fluids during receptive oral sex. Generally these men believed that the chemical agency of saliva and gastric juices neutralized the infectivity of HIV in semen and preseminal fluids. A seropositive man, who was 43-years-old and the head of a nonprofit organization, commented:

> As well versed as I am on this [the safer sex guidelines], I really don't believe that. I mean I just, I can see how contact would occur—bleeding gums or whatever. But the intestinal tract and the salivary, the saliva and everything else that works to break [it] down; it just seems the virus couldn't take that.

The unemployed 24-year-old respondent cited above told us that

> there's nothing wrong with oral sex without a condom. I know that they say you can swallow someone's cum and that kills it automatically in your stomach.

Similarly, a 39-year-old talent agent, who did not know the results of his antibody test, said:

> There's just too many stories about saliva being able to kill the virus, and certainly the digestive juices I believe, would kill the virus.

Several men also believed that the agency of these fluids neutralized HIV during fellatio because ejaculate and preejaculatory fluids contained negligible amounts of the virus. Typical of these was a 23-year-old seronegative executive who thought that preseminal fluids were not a risk factor because

> it's such a negligible amount [the amount of HIV in preejaculatory fluids]. And what's in your mouth is probably gonna kill it first. And well depending upon how you're having the oral sex, there's probably gonna be some air around to kill any little bit that's there.

A few men further defended this belief on the basis of the prevalence of receptive oral sex with ingestion of semen and preseminal fluids among gay men before AIDS. These men felt that the agency of saliva and/or gastric juices must neutralize HIV because most gay men received ejaculate and preejaculatory fluids into their mouths, especially during anonymous encounters, both before and, to a lesser extent, since the epidemic. They reasoned that more gay men would be ill or dead if these fluids did not inhibit HIV, given the ubiquity of this practice. A 33-year-old financial researcher who did not know his test results commented:

> And I've read or heard that the whole process of ingesting semen is different than when you're getting fucked. Because of the saliva, the digestive juices and everything, by the time it gets into the bloodstream it's neutralized.

Later in the interview he added:

> I think you could cum in somebody's mouth or they could cum in my mouth and I don't think that's one of the main modes of transmission because, from what I've viewed throughout my life, in places like the balcony of The Saint or in movie theaters of tea rooms or whatever, sucking was the main sex because it's the easiest and quickest. Then I figure if it were one of the main means, a hell of a lot more people would have it.

The second group felt that the inhibitory agency of either saliva or urethral acid prevented HIV from being transmitted through the urethral opening to the insertive partner during unprotected anal and oral intercourse. Typical of these was a 30-year-old seropositive caterer who told us that the insertor in anal sex was not at risk because the "urethra is too acidic" for HIV to survive. A 36-year-old attorney, who decided not to learn the results of his HIV antibody test, doubted that the amount of saliva present during oral sex was sufficient to transmit the virus through the urethral opening:

> Now it's been my understanding that you can't get it from kissing. Or at least it's not known anyone ever has. And since it appears to me that the amount of saliva that you're exposed to, if someone gives you a blow job, is very very small compared to the amount you get when you're kissing, it seems to me that there's nominal risk.

Excuses

The men offering excuses for unprotected intercourse generally felt that their sexual conduct was risky but attributed their behavior to forces they were unable to control. We organized their responses into four categories of reasons: (a) the influence of drugs and alcohol, (b) sexual passion, (c) emotional needs, and (d) partner coercion.

The influence of drugs or alcohol. The most commonly cited excuse for unprotected sex was the use of drugs or alcohol. Almost all of the respondents offering this excuse insisted that unprotected intercourse was atypical behavior that occurred only when they were "high" or "stoned." These men contended that drugs or alcohol impaired their judgment, lowered their inhibitions, or reduced their ability to resist a partner's urging or pressure to engage in unprotected oral or anal sex.

Characteristic of respondents claiming that insobriety was responsible for unprotected intercourse was a 27-year-old seronegative lawyer. During the interview, this man told us about an episode of unprotected anal sex with a physician. Although the respondent began to put a condom on his penis, the doctor said to the respondent, "No, you don't need that. You're OK." The respondent assumed that the doctor was positive and that, therefore, "it didn't matter to him" if the respondent took the insertive role in anal sex and did not use protection. The respondent said that he then proceeded "to fuck" the physician without a condom because "I was really drunk and not thinking about it." He then added that he "felt sorry about it later."

Similarly, two other men attributed unprotected intercourse to the effects of drugs and alcohol. Both respondents felt that insobriety impaired either their judgment or their will. The first, an untested, 27-year-old graduate student, commented:

> I met this guy and we went home. And ah, I was very drunk. And I don't know whether he was drunk or not. But I did, and I'm not real proud of this, fuck him without a condom. I didn't cum in him, but ah, that was because I was drunk. I shouldn't say that was because I was drunk because I, that sort of abrogates responsibility, but I was.

The second, who was a 30-year-old coordinator of an AIDS information service and seropositive, remarked:

> Ah there was, I was introducing condoms to people and being safe with people I had sex with. Ah, but there was one time I was doing, ah I was doing a lot of cocaine. And I let this guy fuck me, and he wouldn't use a condom. And I asked him to just make sure that he pulled out. And I think he did, or I thought he did, but he might not have because I was high.

Sexual passion. A second frequently offered reason for unprotected intercourse was sexual desire or lust. Nearly all the men offering this excuse felt their behavior was uncharacteristic of them and attributable to uncontrollable urges, which overwhelmed their intent to use protection. These men typically described these urges as powerful biological needs and drives, which they dubbed passion or "horniness." For example, a 29-year-old seropositive consultant told us that he occasionally anally penetrated without a condom two of his regular partners because of "sexual passion." Another, a 24-year-old word processor who was seronegative, sometimes allowed men to ejaculate in his mouth because he didn't "have the willpower to pull away" because he "really wanted it." This same respondent also let "a stranger" anally penetrate him without a condom because he was "so horny" that he lost his "sense of reality" and didn't "think rationally."

Several other men attributed unprotected sexual conduct to overwhelming erotic desires. One respondent, a 26-year-old computer operator who was infected, said:

> The first time we met there was unprotected oral sex. And he is HIV positive. . . . There was unprotected oral sex and unprotected anal sex where he did not cum. . . . And the second time—we've only had sex twice—we had brought condoms, the whole bit. You know what I mean, like we were all ready to go. And you know, somewhere along the course of action we forgot to put, you know, to bring out the condoms. . . . And he did cum inside of me. And you know, we both felt bad, so stupid about it. There hadn't even been drinking. . . . It just happened. It was passion.

Another, who was a 41-year-old seronegative pharmacy supervisor, told us:

> I mean it's you know, sometimes you go with all good intentions. And you say to yourself, "You're not gonna let yourself do this. You're not gonna suck the head. Right!" But you know, you see him with a, you know, big cock in your face, and it's not always easy to say, you know, "No, I'm not gonna do it." It's, you know, there are certain basic instincts I guess that take over. And ah, you can't always be as controlled as you want to be.

And a third, who was a 57-year-old cab driver and seropositive, stated:

> Ah, I know there's one particularly hot guy. Well he, he works in the movies, I guess. Just a stud, you know. Ah, just completely rejecting the idea [of using

a condom during anal sex]. Ah, and so once, we did have a sessio
fucked the hell out of me. And I'm happy to say, he just, he couldn
all. And even thought I was so overwhelmed by the passion of the moment
that I would have permitted him that pleasure, things sort of lucked out, as it
were.

Emotional needs. Some men explained incidents of unprotected sex as
an expression of love, affection, or acceptance. Typically these men
participated in unprotected intercourse to demonstrate their emotional
feelings for their partners who were usually their lovers or boyfriends.
Many described their behavior as a sacrifice made for their partners,
which was attributable to understandable and even altruistic motives.

For example, a 28-year-old waiter who had not been tested engaged in
unprotected oral sex with a regular partner because he really cared for this
partner and viewed the act as "an expression of [his] love for him."
Another man, a 39-year-old model who was seropositive, had unprotected
receptive anal sex with his lover whom he knew was infected because he
wanted to show the lover "that he was going to be loved and nurtured and
all." He stated that he wanted to be sure he did not make the lover "feel
like a pariah." Similarly, a 34-year-old seronegative journalist participated in unprotected insertive anal intercourse, albeit without ejaculation,
with his lover who had AIDS. He told us that he did it because "it was
psychologically for our relationship at that point important."

Partner coercion. Other men claimed that their partners coerced them
into engaging in unprotected intercourse. Generally these men perceived
themselves as victims of either other men's pressure or their deceptive
conduct. They insisted that they intended to use protection but that their
partners undermined their resolve.

There were two subgroups among these respondents. The first included respondents who were pressured into participating in unprotected sex. Typically their partners either refused or urged them not to
use protection. The cab driver quoted above told us that, on the increasingly rare occasions when he did not use a condom, the "problem was
with the other partner," who just "absolutely refused to use condoms."
Another, a 27-year-old man who was untested, insisted that he "went into
a situation saying, 'I'm not . . . there's not going to be any oral-genital
contact here.'" However, he admitted that he often got "weak in [his]
strength" and could not maintain his intent to practice safer sex in the face
of his partner's desire for unprotected fellatio. Finally, a 30-year-old

seropositive graduate student said he stopped seeing his HIV-positive boyfriend because "he forced me to do things sexually that I didn't want to do" such as "sucking him off" and ingesting the semen. The respondent felt that he had been "raped" by the lover and "forced to have sex against [his] will."

The second group consisted of a handful of men who were deceived into having unprotected receptive anal sex. These men usually thought the insertive partner used protection but later discovered that this was not the case. For example, a 23-year-old untested artist's assistant reported he noticed after one instance of receptive anal intercourse that the insertive partner did not use protection. This respondent assumed that the insertor was going to put on a condom before entering his anus because "there was a condom right next to him," that is, on the bedside table.

DISCUSSION

The men's accounts of unprotected sex both embody and constitute social constructions of the risk of HIV transmission during intercourse and culturally available explanations for untoward sexual behavior. In this final section of the chapter, we describe these risk definitions and explanations more broadly, further differentiate men using justifications from those citing excuses, and comment upon the implications of our findings for HIV prevention.

Within the cultural milieu surrounding our respondents, there exist two competing constructions of the risk of HIV transmission associated with unprotected intercourse; they can be labeled the *public health* and the *folk* constructions. The men we interviewed justified or excused their unprotected sexual behavior by drawing upon these risk definitions, applying them to their own situation, and thus revitalizing them as cultural constructions. Our review of public health, HIV prevention, and gay literature indicates that the public health definition emerged shortly after the early (1981-84) epidemiological studies of the risk factors for AIDS and the discovery of HIV in 1984. The folk construction appeared later, following the appearance of epidemiological and laboratory evidence concerning the effect of saliva and gastric juices on HIV and the presence of HIV within preseminal fluids. Both definitions differ in regard to the relative risk of HIV transmission during unprotected anal and oral intercourse.

The public health construction of risk depicts all forms of unprotected oral and anal intercourse as risky unless both partners either had been monogamous from the mid-1970s or had tested seronegative 6 months after their last unsafe encounter (Wofsky 1988). These practices are regarded as risky because they have the potential for transmitting HIV-infected body fluids (blood, saliva, semen, preseminal fluids) directly into the bloodstream through either the urethral opening or tiny lacerations in the skin or linings of the anus, mouth, or genitals (Jaffe and Lifson 1988). The transmission of this virus during intercourse may occur in three distinct ways: First, the thrusting of the penis during anal sex may cause small tears on its surface or in the lining of the anus, which may provide infected body fluids a portal of entry into the bloodstream. Second, periodontal and sexually transmitted diseases, dental flossing and brushing, and deep kissing can create similar cuts or sores on the penis or mouth. During oral intercourse, these lacerations may permit infected body fluids to enter the bloodstream. Third, HIV also can enter the bloodstream during intercourse through the mucous lining of the urethral opening (Koop 1986; Mass 1985).

This construction also holds that there are relative differences in the level of risk associated with anal and oral sex (Jennings 1988). Available epidemiological data indicate that unprotected receptive anal intercourse with ejaculation of semen is the most consistently identified risk behavior for the transmission of HIV throughout the epidemic (Institute of Medicine 1986, 1988; Turner et al. 1989), probably due to the strong likelihood of anal lacerations from penile thrusting (Jennings 1988). However, the risk of infection from unprotected oral-genital relations and unprotected insertive anal intercourse appears to be less. Although several epidemiological studies found no statistical association between oral-genital contact and HIV infection (Lyman et al. 1986; Moss et al. 1987; Detels et al. 1989), a handful of isolated and often unsubstantiated case reports have described infection through receptive oral sex (Wofsky 1988; Jaffe and Lifson 1988). In addition, only a few epidemiological studies have reported statistical relationships between unprotected insertive anal intercourse and HIV infection (Detels et al. 1989). Thus available data seem to indicate that unprotected receptive anal intercourse is a highly efficient means of transmitting HIV, and there is probably less risk of infection through unprotected fellatio and insertive anal intercourse (Institute of Medicine 1986, 1988; Turner et al. 1989; Detels et al. 1989).

Within metropolitan New York, local public health agencies and AIDS organizations have been the principal advocates of the public health definition of risk (Siegel et al. 1986). These groups, which have mounted continuous HIV prevention campaigns aimed at gay and bisexual men, have in their guidelines for safer sex sought to eliminate all HIV transmission risk during intercourse.

Accordingly, although their guidelines often acknowledged different levels of risk for anal and oral sex, they, nevertheless, have recommended the use of condoms during both these practices. In addition, the guidelines promulgated by such gay organizations such as Gay Men's Health Crisis (GMHC) have recommended not taking ejaculate, preejaculatory fluids, or the glans of the penis into the mouth during unprotected receptive fellatio (Gay Men's Health Crisis 1986).

The men we interviewed were quite familiar with the public health construction of risk. As was the case in previous research (Becker and Joseph 1988; Stall et al. 1988), our respondents spoke knowingly about the public health model of HIV transmission and prevention. Many reported learning about this model from reading articles in the gay and mainstream press, attending GMHC or the Body Positive's (an organization serving seropositive individuals) workshops and forums, and talking to friends and community health activists and practitioners.

The accounts cited in the interviews partly drew upon the public health construction of risk. Many of our respondents justified engaging in unprotected intercourse on the grounds that they avoided the conditions the public health model of transmission specified as necessary for the transmission of HIV. Some defended their behavior on the basis of medical evidence that they or their partners were not infected, usually based on a negative result on the HIV-antibody test. Others rationalized their behavior on the grounds that they followed the guidelines for safe unprotected receptive fellatio. Typically these men claimed that they did not take the glans of the penis into their mouths and thus avoided ingesting semen or preseminal fluids during receptive oral sex.

The folk construction asserts a different model of HIV infection and prevention during intercourse. According to this definition, the transmission of HIV requires the passage of infected blood or semen directly into the bloodstream through lacerations either on the penis or on the interior lining of the mouth or anus. Unlike the public health construction, the folk model regards preejaculatory fluids and the urethral opening as ineffective transmitters of HIV. The model maintains that laboratory findings provide no conclusive evidence that preseminal fluids contain HIV and also indicate that the chemical agency of saliva and gastric juices neutralize the infectivity of the virus (Jennings 1988, pp. 53-59; Fox et al. 1988). Hence, the chances of viral infection through the urethral opening during oral sex are minimal.

This construction also perceives wide differences in the relative risk of anal and oral intercourse. In this definition, unprotected receptive anal sex with ejaculation constitutes the only form of intercourse proven to be risky. The failure of epidemiological studies to demonstrate a consistent relationship between HIV infection and insertive anal sex and/or oral-genital contact indicates, according to this construction, that it is highly unlikely that these acts effectively transmit the virus. In addition, the documented inhibitory effect of saliva on the infectivity of HIV almost completely diminishes the risk of transmission during fellatio.

The folk construction also uses medical and social indicators to discern the HIV status of potential sexual partners. The determination of this status is based on medical tests for the presence of antibodies to HIV and for immune functioning as well as social evidence of illness, promiscuity, or a high-risk past (Communication Technologies 1987; Valdiserri et al. 1987). Men are presumed to be infected if they test seropositive, have low T-cell counts, look unhealthy, engage in anonymous sex, have sexual histories of high-risk behavior, or come from areas with a high prevalence of the disease.

Many of our respondents' accounts of unprotected intercourse embod-ied the folk construction. Most of the men justified participating in unprotected intercourse on the grounds that they avoided the conditions specified in the folk model of transmission as necessary for the transmis-sion of HIV. Many defended their behavior on the basis of social evidence of seronegativity—either a sexual background or a geographic locale that could be characterized as low risk. Other men rationalized engaging in unprotected oral sex on the basis of avoiding the exchange of either semen and/or preseminal fluids. Typically these men felt that their behavior was safe because they did not ingest fluids that could potentially contain HIV. Others justified acts of unprotected insertive anal intercourse and fellatio on the grounds that there were no lacerations, which they believed precluded transmission of the virus. Finally, some men defended partici-pating in unprotected insertive anal sex and oral-genital relations on the basis of the chemical agency of saliva, gastric juices, and urethral acid, which they felt killed or inhibited the infectivity of HIV.

The accounts cited in the interviews also reflected culturally available explanations for problematic erotic conduct. Within the broader culture, there are a set of socially legitimate reasons for engaging in improper sexual behavior (Luker 1975). Typically these explanations affirm the validity of normative expectations but attempt to neutralize reputational damage by denying the risk of discovery, pregnancy, or disease as well as individual responsibility for participating in the act. That is, they assert that the act was wrong but maintain that there was almost no chance of either being found out or becoming pregnant or sick and attribute responsibility for this behavior to situations and forces that were usually out of the individual's control, such as insobriety, lust, affection, pleasure, or duress (Masters, Johnson, & Kolodny 1982).

The justifications and excuses reported by our respondents incorporated these explanations. Generally, the men offering justifications defended their behavior on the grounds that there was no risk of becoming infected. In addition, respondents citing excuses blamed their behavior on insobriety, sexual passion, emotional needs, and coercion.

These constructions also account for some of the attitudinal, emotional, and behavioral differences observed among respondents offering excuses and justifications. The men citing justifications usually accepted either the public health or the folk definition of risk. Consequently, these men believed that unprotected intercourse was safe in the absence of infectivity, ejaculation, lacerations, or insertion of the penile glans into the mouth. Hence, the men rarely expressed regret or guilt about their own episodes of unprotected sex that occurred in the absence of these conditions. They felt their behavior was safe and conformed to normative expectations within the gay community, calling for the avoidance of risk during intercourse. It is not surprising that the men knowingly and frequently engaged in unprotected intercourse with multiple partners when they perceived that the conditions existed to make such practices safe.

Alternately, respondents offering excuses usually accepted the public health construction of risk. Consequently, these men believed that unprotected intercourse was always risky unless it occurred between two men who both tested seronegative for HIV antibodies. Hence, the men frequently expressed regret, guilt, or remorse for participating in unprotected sex, which they often regarded as "irresponsible," "stupid," or "wrong" behavior. (By acknowledging these feelings, they appeared to be trying to soften the reactions of others—in this case, the interviewer and/or research team—to their disclosure of normative violation.) Moreover, these men generally described their episodes of unprotected intercourse as isolated and unintended relapses from their normal pattern of safer sex, usually resulting from insobriety, sexual passion, emotional need, or coercion.

The accounts cited in the interviews have implications for HIV prevention. Most prevention campaigns have sought to induce compliance with safer sex guidelines among gay and bisexual men by both raising individuals' levels of knowledge about practices implicated in HIV transmission and creating a normative expectation within the gay community that men will practice only safer sex. Although these strategies have been somewhat effective, the explanations offered by the men in our study for participation in unprotected intercourse suggest that there are several additional factors to be considered. First, in the absence of compelling epidemiological/scientific data about the risk of transmission associated with insertive anal sex and oral-genital relations, men draw conclusions about the relative risk inherent in those behaviors from experimentally acquired folk constructions. Efforts must be made either to clarify the level of risk associated with these practices or, in the meantime, to emphasize their uncertain safety rather than their uncertain risk.

Second, gay men are making various assumptions in evaluating the risk inherent in a given sexual encounter that are likely to be highly unreliable. For example, men are appraising the likelihood that a potential partner is infected based on the partner's unsubstantiated reports of prior behavior, past level of sexual activity, and past locales of that activity. Prevention efforts must stress the poor and unreliable predictive value of these folk definitions of risk status.

Finally, sexual activity is a highly charged, interpersonal mix of physical pleasure and complex psychological states. Accordingly, persuasion or coercion, physical attraction or desire, and emotional bonds or needs exert a powerful influence over erotic conduct. For example, the influence of a sexual partner can undermine an individual's intent to practice safer sex and prompt him to engage in risky conduct. Similarly, the powerful drives associated with love, affection, and desire can foster further episodes of risk behavior. These intense interpersonal dynamics will be difficult to influence solely through education and normative change and may instead require interventions that focus on enhancing skills in interpersonal dynamics.

REFERENCES

Becker, Marshall H. and Jill G. Joseph. 1988. "AIDS and Behavioral Change to Reduce Risk: A Review." *American Journal of Public Health* 78:394-410.

Coates, Thomas J. 1990. "Strategies for Modifying Sexual Behavior for Primary and Secondary Prevention of HIV Disease." *Journal of Consulting and Clinical Psychology* 58:57-69.

Coates, Thomas J., Ron D. Stall, Joseph A. Catania, and Susan M. Kegeles. 1988. "Behavioral Factors in the Spread of HIV Infection." *AIDS* 2(Suppl.):S239-45.

Communication Technologies. 1987. *Designing an Effective AIDS Prevention Campaign Strategy for San Francisco: Results From the Fourth Probability Sample of an Urban Gay Male Community.* San Francisco: San Francisco AIDS Foundation.

Connell, R. W., June Crawford, Susan Kippay, G. W. Dowsett, Don Baxter, and Lex Watson. 1989. "Facing the Epidemic: Changes in the Sexual Lives of Gay and Bisexual Men in Australia and Their Implications for AIDS Prevention Strategies." *Social Problems* 36:384-402.

Detels, Roger, Patricia English, Barbara R. Visscher, Lisa Jacobson, Lawrence A. Kingsley, Joan S. Chmiel, Janice P. Dudley, Lois J. Eldred, and Harold M. Ginzburg. 1989. "Serocoversion, Sexual Activity, and Condom Use Among 2915 HIV Seronegative Men Followed for up to 2 Years." *Journal of Acquired Immune Deficiency Syndromes* 2:77-83.

Fox, P.C., A. Wolff, C. K. Yeh, et al. 1988. "Salvia Inhibits HIV-1 Infectivity." *Journal of the American Dental Association* 116:635-7.

Gay Men's Health Crisis. 1986. *An Ounce of Prevention Is Worth a Pound of Cure: Safer Sex Guidelines for Gay and Bisexual Men.* New York: Gay Men's Health Crisis.

Institute of Medicine. 1986. *Confronting AIDS: Update 1988.* Washington, DC: National Academy Press.

————. 1988. *Confronting AIDS: Directions for Public Health, Health Care, and Research.* Washington, DC: National Academy Press.

Jaffe, Harold W. and Alan R. Lifson. 1988. "Acquisition and Transmission of HIV." Pp. 19-27 in *The Medical Management of AIDS.* Edited by M. A. Sande and P. A. Volberding. Phildelphia: W. B. Saunders.

Jennings, Chris. 1988. *Understanding and Preventing Aids: A Book for Everyone.* Cambridge, MA: Health Alert Press.

Judson, Franklin N. 1977. "Sexually Transmitted Disease in Gay Men." *Sexually Transmitted Diseases* 4:76-78.

Martin, John L. 1987. "The Impact of AIDS on Gay Male Sexual Behavior Patterns in New York City." *American Journal of Public Health* 77:578-81.

Koop, C. Everett. 1986 *Surgeon General's Report on Acquired Immune Deficiency Syndrome.* Washington, DC: U.S. Department of Health.

Luker, Kristine. 1975. *Taking Chances.* Berkeley: University of California Press.

Lyman, David, Warren Winkelstein, Michael Ascher, and Jay A. Levy. 1986. "Minimal Risk of AIDS-Associated Retrovirus Infection by Oral Genital Contact." *Journal of the American Medical Association.* 255:1703.

Martin, John L., Laura Dean, Mark Garcia, and William Hall. 1989. "The Impact of AIDS on a Gay Community: Changes in Sexual Behavior, Substance Abuse, and Mental Health." *American Journal of Community Psychology.* 17:269-293.

Masters, William H., Virginia E Johnson, and Robert C. Kolodny. 1982. *Human Sexuality.* Boston: Little, Brown.

Mass, Lawrence. 1985. *Medical Answers About AIDS.* New York: Gay Men's Health Crisis.

McKusick, Leon, William Hortsman, and Thomas J. Coates. 1985. "AIDS and Sexual Behavior Reported by Gay Men in San Francisco." *American Journal of Public Health* 75:493-96.

McKusick, Leon, James A. Wiley, Thomas J. Coates, Ronald Stall, Glen Saika, Stephen Morin, Kenneth Charles, William Hortsman, and Marrus A. Conant. 1985. "Reported Changes in the Sexual Behavior of Men at Risk for AIDS, San Francisco, 1982-84: The AIDS Behavioral Research Project." *U.S. Public Health Reports* 100:622-29.

Merton, Robert K., Marjorie Fiske, and Patricia L. Kendall. 1956. *The Focused Interview.* New York: Free Press.

Moss, Andrew R., Dennis Osmond, Peter Bacchetti, Jean Claude Chermann, Francoise Barre-Sinoussi, and James Carlson. 1987. "Risk Factors for AIDS and HIV Seropositivity in Homosexual Men." *American Journal of Epidemiology* 125:1035-1047.

Ross, Michael W. 1988a. "Attitudes Towards Condoms as AIDS Prophylaxis in Homosexual Men: Dimensions and Measurement." *Psychology and Health* 2:291-99.

———. 1988b. "Personality Factors That Differentiate Homosexual Men With Positive and Negative Attitudes Toward Condom Use." *New York State Journal of Medicine* 88: 626-28.

———. 1988c. "Relationship of Combinations of AIDS Counseling and Testing to Safer Sex and Condom Use in Homosexual Men." *Community Health Studies* 12:322-27.

Scott, Marvin and Stanford Lyman. 1968. "Accounts." *American Sociological Review* 33:46-62.

Siegel, Karolynn, Laurie J. Bauman, Grace H. Christ, and Susan Krown. 1988a. "Patterns of Change in Sexual Behavior Among Gay Men in New York City." *Archives of Sexual Behavior* 17:481-97.

Siegel, Karolynn, Phyllis B. Grodsky, and A. Herman. 1986. "AIDS Risk Reduction Guidelines: A Review and Analysis." *Journal of Community Health* 11:235-43.

Siegel, Karolynn, Frances Mesagno, Jin-Yi Chen, and Grace Christ. 1988b. "Factors Distinguishing Homosexual Males Practicing Risky and Safer Sex." *Social Science and Medicine* 28:561-69.

Stall, Ron, Thomas Coates, and Charles Hoff. 1988. "Behavioral Risk Reduction for HIV Infection Among Gay and Bisexual Men: A Review of Results From the United States." *American Psychologist* 43:878-85.

Stall, Ron, Leon McKusick, James Wiley, Thomas J. Coates, and David G. Ostrow. 1986. "Alcohol and Drug Use During Sexual Activity and Compliance With Safe Sex Guidelines for AIDS: The AIDS Behavioral Research Project" *Health Education Quarterly* 13:359-71.

Turner, Charles F., Heather G. Miller, and Lincoln Moses, 1989. *AIDS: Sexual Behavior and Intravenous Drug Use.* Washington, DC: National Academy Press.

Valdiserri, Ronald O., David W. Lyter, Lawrence A. Kingsley, Laura C. Leviton, Janet W. Schofield, James Huggins, Monto Ho, and Charles R. Rinaldo. 1987. "The Effect of Group Education on Improvising Attitudes About AIDS Risk Reduction." *New York State Journal of Medicine* 87:272-78.

Valdiserri, Ronald O., David Lyter, Laura Leviton, Catherine M. Callahan, Lawrence A. Kingsley, and Charles R. Rinaldo. 1988. "Variables Influencing Condom Use in a Cohort of Gay and Bisexual Men." *American Journal of Public Health* 78:801-5.

Williams, Daniel C. 1979. "Sexually Transmitted Diseases in Gay Men: An Insider's View." *Sexually Transmitted Diseases* 6:278-80.

Wofsky, Constance B. 1988. "Prevention of HIV Transmission." Pp. 29-43 in *The Medical Management of AIDS.* Edited by M. A. Sande and P. A. Volberding. Philadelphia: W. B. Saunders.

4

Women Don't Wear Condoms:
AIDS Risk Among Sexual Partners
of IV Drug Users

Laurie Wermuth
Jennifer Ham
Rebecca L. Robbins

Women sexual partners of intravenous (IV) drug users must cope with uncertainty and lack of control when they address their risk for AIDS. They lack complete knowledge about their male partners' needle use and sexual practices and their partners' HIV-antibody test taking and results. In addition, women lack direct control over the preventive remedy offered to women by public health authorities—the condom— that requires the active cooperation of their male partners. Compared with gay men, the numbers of infected women are still small, but the recent increases are frightening.

Although the majority of female AIDS cases in the United States are attributed to IV drug use, the percentage attributed to sexual transmission is rising, more than doubling from 14% in 1982 to 31% in 1989. During the period of April 1988 to March 1989, there were 628 cases of sexual

AUTHORS' NOTE: This work was supported by a grant (MH4259) from the National Institute of Mental Health and the National Institute on Drug Abuse. We would like to thank our colleagues for their comments: Sarah Derby, Hsiao-ti Falcone, Mindy Fullilove, David R. Gibson, Joseph Guydish, Stephen Hulley, Renata Kiefer, Jane Lovelle-Drache, Thomas Murphy, and James Sorensen. Address correspondence to Laurie Wermuth, Department of Sociology and Social Work, California State University, Chico, CA 95929-0445.

transmission to women from IV drug users, a jump from 380 cases during the previous year (Centers for Disease Control 1989a, 1989b, 1990). For women with infected partners, the risk of acquiring an HIV infection increases with repeated sexual exposures but is lower if condoms are used (Hearst and Hulley 1988). In addition, AIDS risk in sex is compounded by other dangers: If women do not already use IV drugs, they may be introduced to the practice by their male partners (Rosenbaum 1981; Zahn and Ball 1974; O'Donnell, Besteman, and Jones 1967), and, if they are infected and become pregnant, their infants are at risk for HIV infection.

Models of health-related behaviors based upon individualistic conceptions of risk may be inadequate to address the problem of the sexual transmission of HIV. Risk reduction models developed for smoking or other health-related behaviors are not necessarily applicable to women sexual partners of men at high risk for HIV infection. These models emphasize the individual's "health beliefs" (Becker 1974), self-efficacy (Bandura 1977), and motivations and skills to implement changes (Joseph, Montgomery, Kessler, Ostlow, and Wortmen 1988). The health belief and self-efficacy frameworks capture the cognitive process of individuals changing their behaviors but neglect other important determinants, such as less-than-conscious emotional factors, interpersonal relationships, and social context. Most striking is the lack of causal weight given to partners in sexual activity and drug injection (Des Jarlais, Friedman, and Strug 1986). Even when a long list of variables is included (Catania, Kegeles, and Coates 1990; Coates, Stall, Catania, and Kegeles 1988), determinants of risk practices based on the partner's behavior or the couple relationship may not be discovered. Models that include values and expectations may be more successful in predicting who will adopt condom use (Kegeles, Adler, and Irwin 1989) but may not discover determinants beyond those values and expectations.

This chapter offers a profile of risk for 77 women sexual partners of IV drug users and describes the strategies by which they manage their risk for HIV infection. The discussion and conclusion sections elaborate the implications of those strategies for AIDS prevention and research efforts.

DESCRIPTION OF STUDY AND RESPONDENTS

This discussion is based upon 77 baseline interviews conducted with women sexual partners of IV drug users in the San Francisco Bay Area. Criteria for entry to the study were not having used IV drugs in the past

6 months and having had sex during the past year with a man who had used IV drugs since 1978. Women currently injecting drugs were excluded and referred to a parallel study of IV drug users (Gibson, Wermuth, Lovelle-Drache, Ham, and Sorensen 1989) so that this study could maintain its focus on risk for sexual transmission. Study participants were located through newspaper ads, distribution of fliers to medical and drug treatment clinics, other research projects, chain referral, and individuals entering the methadone detoxification program at San Francisco General Hospital. Questionnaire items included demographic characteristics, sexual practices, partners' needle-use practices, HIV-testing history of self and partners, and questions about relationships. The latter part of the interview consisted of open-ended questions, including items about the woman's perceived risk, how her partner's drug use affected her, and hypothetical questions regarding condom use and her relationship.

Respondents

Selected characteristics of the respondents are listed in Table 4.1. Half were between the ages of 30 and 40 years, with the average being 33 and the range from 19 to 57 years old. Of the women, 40 were white, 28 black, 7 Hispanic, and 1 Native American. Most were in an ongoing relationship with an IV drug user and had few other sexual partners: 45 were married or living with a partner, 49 had had only one sexual partner in the past 30 days, and 63 reported three or fewer sexual partners during the previous year. Although 9 of the women reported being involved in their current relationships for less than 12 months, 32 of the women had been with their partners from 1 to 3 years, and 22 reported a length of relationship from 4 to 9 years. An additional 14 had been involved for over 10 years. Of the 77 women, 61 had children and 54 had at least a high school education or GED; 25 were employed full or part time, and 30 received public assistance (AFDC, GA, or SSI). As a group, respondents were relatively knowledgeable about AIDS, with the majority scoring above or at the average score of 80% correct answers.

The methods for locating respondents required that women contact the project after hearing about it through one of the channels listed above. We had only a few opportunities to actively recruit women to the study; most of those discussions occurred in our home-base methadone clinic. Most of the 77 women who participated were married to or living with their sexual partners, had few other sexual partners, and appeared by their high

Table 4.1 Characteristics of Women Sexual Partners of IV Drug Users (N = 77)

Characteristics	Percentage
Perceived risk for AIDS	64
Sociodemographics:	
age—below 30	31
between 30 and 40	51
40 or older	18
white (versus nonwhite)	52
married or living with partner	59
relationship with partner 4 years or longer	47
have children	79
high school degree or GED	70
employed full or part time	33
injected drugs since 1978	47
Male partners' needle practices:	
partner injected drugs in past year	75
partner shared needles in last year	48
partner currently cleaning needles always or uses sterile needles	31
Sexual practices:	
had sexual intercourse in past 30 days	73
only 1 sexual partner in past 30 days	64
had fewer than 4 sexual partners in past year	82
HIV-antibody testing:	
woman never tested	40
woman tested positive	3
partner's testing status unknown/never been tested	53
partner tested positive	11
AIDS knowledge: subjects scoring average or better	64

NOTE: Percentages have been rounded.

rates of HIV-antibody testing to be relatively motivated to protect themselves from HIV infection. High testing rates may also be due in part to location, because AIDS services and information are widely available in San Francisco. In addition, the high proportion of high school graduates suggests the sample underselected for the poorest and most socially marginal among women sexual partners of IV drug users. Women in the sex industry were underrepresented in part due to screening out active IV drug users (who often exchange sex for money or drugs). Only two respondents reported sufficiently high numbers of sexual partners to suggest current prostitution activities, although it is possible that there were additional steady relationships in which sex was traded for drugs, housing, or cash. The women by and large did not have many sexual partners: 70 of the 77 women in the study had five or fewer partners in the last year and 47 had only one sexual partner in the past year.

Risk for AIDS

Despite some bias toward a motivated group, respondents' relationships with their partners appeared to pose considerable risk: 58 of the women had partners who had injected drugs during the past year and a considerable proportion (37 out of 77) of those men shared needles as well. An additional 6 women were uncertain about partners' needle-sharing practices. Only 24 reported their partners to be using new or sterilized needles. In addition, despite the exclusion criterion, 2 women were currently injecting drugs and many others were at risk for relapse (Stimmel, Goldberg, Rotkopf, and Cohen 1977; Gearing 1974) because nearly half of the women had injected drugs since 1978.

The majority of the women had already been HIV-antibody tested when they entered the study. Half of the women reported that their partners had been tested, but an additional 10 women did not know whether their partners had been tested. Two women reported themselves to be HIV infected, and 8 reported their male partners to be infected.

More than half of the respondents demonstrated high knowledge about transmission and methods for preventing HIV infection but relatively few reported using condoms: 46 had never used condoms in their current relationships; 23 women reported some to consistent condom use. Couples in which the man was known to be HIV infected were far more likely to use condoms. Of the 23 women reporting condom use, 7 had partners who were known to be HIV infected and 7 additional couples had already been using condoms for birth control. The majority of couples were sexually active, with 56 reporting intercourse during the past 30 days.

COPING WITH RISK FOR AIDS:
STRATEGIES FOR MANAGING
UNCERTAINTY AND LACK OF CONTROL

Implicit in the model of individual risk reduction based on health beliefs is the assumption that, when faced with a noncompliant partner, the highly motivated individual chooses not to engage in risky sexual activity. Although seemingly reasonable, this formulation gives insufficient causal weight to the interpersonal, social, and material constraints on such choices. Assumptions of individually driven decision making may be more valid for casual encounters in which there are no fears of reprisal or other serious costs for refused sex; but when individuals do not have equal "bargaining power" in relationships, this assumption may not apply (Worth 1989; Collins 1974). Especially in longer-term and marital relationships in which there is greater personal investment, individuals consider the possible loss of the relationship that pressing for change could bring.

Factors of social class, gender inequalities, race/ethnicity, and the stigma of being partner to a drug addict converge to enhance the danger of AIDS among this group of women (Fullilove et al. forthcoming; Worth 1989). Poor women are constrained in their choices about relationships and living situations in ways that middle-class women are not, and they may not experience the freedom to regulate sexual practices or to separate from men. Concerns regarding food, shelter, and care of their children may overshadow worries about AIDS (Mays and Cochran 1988) and, when addiction is added to these factors, risk is especially high. Warnings about AIDS are likely to be overshadowed by risk of violence, by withdrawal discomforts, and by efforts to maintain housing and care for children.

Cultural values that place a premium on male prerogative in relationships also constrain women's choices. Especially among less acculturated Hispanic couples, for example, it is not acceptable for women to bring up the topic of sexual relations or to propose practices such as using condoms. Consequently, it is problematic for women to be assertive in protecting themselves from possible HIV infection.

Additional factors contribute to risk. Women sexual partners of IV drug users are a privatized group; many are secretive about their partners' drug use and isolated from those who could encourage them to take protective

measures. Some women do not know that their sexual partners have injected drugs. Emotional and cognitive factors also may impede women's
abilities to address the risks they face. A common interpretation of
women's seeming indifference to their AIDS risk is that they are "in
denial" and, in the vocabulary of the 12-step self-help programs, are
"coaddicts." Their continued relationships with drug users are seen as
complicity with the pathological behavior of their partners. Although
there may be a disproportionate number of overly dependent relationships
among these couples, it is also possible that women downplay their HIV
risk much as people generally downplay the chances of becoming victims
of negative life events (Siegel and Gibson 1988; Weinstein 1980, 1982).

How do women cope with the situation of knowing they may be at risk
for HIV infection yet not experience direct control over the remedies to
that situation? Our interviews revealed that women devised varied and
multiple strategies to reduce uncertainty and increase control over their
risk. These were not perfect solutions to their HIV risk, but they often
reduced uncertainty and most often the chances of infection as well.

Talking with Partners

At entry to the study, half of the women had either talked about AIDS
risk and condoms or used them with their partner in the past month. But,
despite the substantial number of couples that had recently talked about
condoms, few agreements to use them resulted. Negotiations raised sensitive issues of loyalty, trust, control, and sexual performance—issues that
threatened to affect the status quo in relationships and cause major
disruptions. In addition, because men with drug or alcohol dependencies
have higher rates of sexual dysfunction (Cocores, Pottash, Gold, and
Miller 1988), proposing condom use could threaten to exacerbate those
difficulties and trigger volatile responses. For example, nine women who
had raised the issue of condoms mentioned that their partners accused
them of having AIDS. Negotiating condom use with partners proved to
be more than a matter of "communication skills." Even when women
made persuasive arguments and stated their wishes assertively, their male
partners did not necessarily agree to use condoms. (In the following
examples, respondents' names have been replaced with fictitious ones.)

Molly's partner reacted angrily to the suggestion that he use condoms:
"What do you think I am, a punk?" He saw a brochure for AIDS testing
at her apartment and quizzed her about it. Molly responded, " 'Well, to be
truthful, I know you are a drug user and you hang out on Polk Street—you

told me that yourself.' I said, 'so why wouldn't I be going in [to be tested].' He really got upset about that."

Jamie proposed to her husband that they use condoms and repeated the request several times, but he consistently refused. Jamie told the interviewer that she was "gonna keep trying" to get her husband to cooperate. When asked about a hypothetical situation involving their using condoms, she answered, "It would depend on if he was drunk. . . . If he wasn't drunk, maybe he would understand, but if he was drunk there would be a big fight." When asked about difficulties in protecting herself from HIV, however, she did not mention her husband's resistance to condom use but identified her husband's drug use as the key obstacle.

Susan attempted without success to persuade her partner to use condoms: "We talked about AIDS. . . . I don't know, I guess it's an ego thing with him. I tell him it's for our safety and he believes that, but still, he's not ready to [use condoms]." Later in the interview she continued,

> This relationship is the first time I brought up the subject [of using condoms], no matter how painful. I even told him that I did not want to see him anymore. . . . [Separation] worked for a long time . . . it has really made me take a look at what I think of myself, my own self-esteem, and what I am willing to do to stand up for myself.

Despite this woman's assertiveness and communication skills, she was not able to get her partner to practice safer sex; instead, they had sex less often.

Talking and even consistent condom use did not necessarily eliminate worry about AIDS. This was especially true for the women who knew their partners were infected. Patricia, whose husband was infected, described her situation:

> I practice safe sex. It's scary, there is no other way to put it. We don't discuss me getting the virus unless a condom breaks. However, we did discuss it this morning because he was telling me it's been a while since I've been tested and I should be tested. I was telling him that I'm not ready for being tested. I'm not looking forward to going through the anxiety and I'm certainly not ready to hear positive results.

Testing of Self and Partner

Testing may be one of the few actions women have direct control over in heterosexual HIV infection risk. HIV-antibody testing was a resource for women who chose to consciously acknowledge risk and wait out the results. Willingness to be tested indicated some acknowledgement of risk and required a waiting time to receive test results, often two weeks or longer. All those who had been tested except two had received negative results. Testing had its shortcomings as a preventive strategy, however. It may have encouraged some women to maintain cautious behavior, but, for others, a negative test result fueled a system of denial in which risky sex and drug use was rationalized.

When women encouraged their partners to be tested, men's reactions varied from anger to gratitude. If the partner tested negative and claimed not to be engaged in needle sharing, then the woman might be somewhat confident that she was safe. However, because of the high rate of relapse among IV drug users and the lack of certainty in partners' reports of needle use and sexual practices, HIV-antibody testing sometimes provided a false sense of security or continued worry.

From women's reports at entry to the study, 47 out of 77 had been tested for HIV antibodies with 2 women reporting having tested positive. Half reported that their partners had been tested; 8 of those reported their male partners to be infected. An additional 10 did not know whether their partners had been tested. Other partners may have been infected and not known it, and some may have known and not told their women partners.

Testing often was used as a conscious, rational strategy to assess current HIV status and to sustain motivation. For women confident that their partners were monogamous and not injecting drugs, HIV-antibody testing provided reassurance that they were presently free from risk. Marianna reported: "I was very concerned when I understood the connection between [AIDS and IV drug use]. But since he stopped using [heroin] and he has had tests, I am not too concerned about it now." However, she continued to fear relapse, as did other women in long relationships with IV drug users. Marianna continued, "Although . . . if he would ever get involved again it would be a very difficult situation because he probably wouldn't tell me about it first . . . so, it feels like there is some danger although it seems to have resolved itself for the moment." To lessen her worry, Marianna asked that her husband tell her right away if he started injecting drugs again. For another woman, Francine, testing for herself and her husband was part of an overall plan to protect herself. Her husband now used only his own "outfit" (needle and syringe), and Francine cleaned his needles once a week when she did the housework.

When women tried and could not get their partners to use condoms, testing at least provided some sense of confidence that the couple had avoided infection thus far. Having one's partner get tested was not always simple. Katherine reported,

> He was open to having [an antibody test], but he works an erratic work schedule and Planned Parenthood's [schedule] wasn't able to coincide with his. So, it ended up that only I got it done. And we both pretty much figured that if I was OK, so was he, since we've been monogamous for 2 years. So we were hoping that that little bit of chance didn't exist with us.

Katherine downplayed the fact that her partner could be infected and that, over time, her chances of infection would increase with repeated sexual exposures (Padian et al. 1987).

Testing also could be posed as a condition for continuing a relationship. Alison became aware of her risk during the course of her pregnancy, when HIV-antibody testing was recommended by her health care providers. She reported,

> It really started to concern me when I was halfway through my pregnancy. I told him, "you're gonna have a test and that's the only way I'm going to resume any relationship after I have the baby. . . . You think I'm joking but I'm serious." I would repeat it from time to time to let him know that I meant it.

A few women combined continued-risk taking behaviors (occasional IV drug use, needle sharing, or unprotected sex) with testing at regular 6-month intervals. These women were IV drug users in methadone maintenance treatment who had reduced practices that put them at risk for HIV but occasionally still engaged in those practices. Testing appeared to be their way to periodically monitor whether they had escaped infection.

Influencing Partners' Needle Practices

Women attempted to influence male partners' drug-use practices to reduce risk and uncertainty. When asked generally about AIDS risk and involvement in their partners' drug habit, approximately a fifth of the women mentioned activities that indicated their influence in "domesticating" their partner's drug use. Within this category were activities women undertook to keep partners' drug use closer to home, a more solitary activity, and one that could be monitored. Nine women reported cleaning their partners' needles or finding a supply of sterile needles; two reported supplying bleach for cleaning needles; and four reported educating their partners about AIDS risk. Many women mentioned their role in stopping or curtailing their partners' risky needle-use practices. Some women encouraged their partners to apply for methadone treatment or to stop using entirely. One woman enlisted the support of local dealers in her efforts, requesting that they first speak to her before selling heroin to her husband. The number of women reporting domesticating activities was relatively small but might have been much greater if we had asked specifically about such endeavors.

In many cases, the domestication strategy fit an existing caretaking role on the part of the woman. Women pressured partners to use drugs less and to limit their social contacts with other drug users. When partners currently were not injecting drugs, women sometimes threatened to leave the relationship or withhold sex if drug injecting was resumed. Eleanor undertook a campaign to educate her husband about his AIDS risk. She convinced him to inject drugs only at home, but she was afraid he would "use" when he was out with his friends. "I was so worried about this . . . that I put the [small bleach] bottles in the glove compartment of the car, thinking if [he shot up he might] have enough sense to run outside and get the bottle of bleach." Susan also became instrumental in her partner's drug-use habits.

> I make sure he has a bottle of bleach whenever he is going out to do something that day. [I tell him] "even though you have your own needle, take the bleach because there is always somebody who doesn't have a needle and they are going to want to use yours."

Georgia pressured her husband to be careful in his drug-use practices, combining vigilance with trust:

> My husband and I have discussed it and now he doesn't share his needles, he cleans them out. . . . The thought is there, it's always there. . . . I keep an eye on him and watch what he does so he doesn't infect me. I am sure that he doesn't mess around with other women, so I am not concerned about that. It's only the needles. I have no choice but to trust him enough to think about me and his son.

Domestication most likely reduced men's risky needle practices and, in turn, women's risk for HIV infection. Partners' safer needle practices or cessation of drug use were more likely than condoms to be the woman's or the couple's focus for eliminating AIDS risk. It seemed that, in these relationships, exercising influence over partners' drug-use practices, and even outside sexual partners, was more familiar and acceptable terrain than negotiation over condom use. Pressures and requests regarding drug use and other partners may have raised tensions and distrust but did not threaten the status quo as could the more vulnerable area of renegotiating the couple's own sexual relationship.

Sizing Up the Costs and Benefits of Pressing for Condom Use

Before introducing the subject of condom use to their partners, women weighed the possible costs and benefits of such a move. This process appeared to parallel processes described for contraceptive decision making (Luker 1975) and for decisions about whether to have an abortion (Smetana and Adler 1979). Women weighed the possibilities in light of their own attitudes and beliefs about proposing condom use and in light of the attitudes of their partners (Ajzen and Fishbein 1973). To understand what the women in the study did to try to negotiate condom use, we asked an open-ended question: "What do you think your partner's reaction would be if you suggested that he always used condoms?" In a preliminary analysis with 65 respondents, 13 had already experienced negative reactions from their partners regarding condom use and an additional 19 anticipated negative reactions (Wermuth and Ham 1989). In later analysis including all 77 women, 23 responses included the prediction of angry or violent responses, 30 included refusals to wear condoms, and 7 included the statement that "she was crazy" to suggest condom use. In addition, individual women reported responses such as ending the relationship and a partner throwing away or ripping up condoms to prevent their use. Negative dispositions toward condom use, and some women's own ambivalence, discouraged pursuit of the issue. Women may have feared losing their relationships if they pushed too hard for condom use.

Changing Relationships or Leaving Relationships

As noted above, the majority of women in the study were in relatively long-term relationships. This no doubt made it more difficult to change entrenched patterns or to leave relationships. Women sometimes found they could not exert influence over their partners' drug-using behavior or partners' other sexual relationships. In response to this, 12 of the women reported leaving relationships due to AIDS risk. An additional 18 stated that they had made changes in their sexual relationship because of AIDS risk. Changes included abstinence or the withholding of sex until risky needle-use behavior was changed, the use of condoms until antibody test results were received, monogamy, and increasing safer sex practices (for example, eliminating oral sex with ejaculation and increasing the use of mutual masturbation).

Gloria used the sex-avoidance strategy. She knew she was at risk because she had witnessed her partner sharing needles with his friends and, when she presented him with condoms, he told her to "just throw them away." Gloria believed that avoiding sexual relationships with drug users was her solution to AIDS risk. She explained to the interviewer,

> That's the reason why we haven't had sex for the last month, because I know what he thinks about the condom and everything . . . we argue and fight when we do any change. I don't know how he'd react if I told him to put one on. We've been together 7 years and he's never had one on.

AIDS risk also moved some women to make greater demands of loyalty on their sexual partners, but such demands did not necessarily result in monogamous relationships. Carlie reported,

> He has an old lady that's staying with him. I told him if I ever catch anything it would be a big problem . . . he likes to have sex with me a whole lot. Every now and then he might give somebody drugs just to go to bed with them. . . . I tell him I don't want him messin' around with too many people.

Andrea espoused sexual loyalty, but she herself was not monogamous: "I don't have a lot of sex partners. I mess with one man that I know is going to be only messin' with me. . . . I don't have no man that's been messin' around with no other woman."

Among the 33 women in the study who had recent histories of IV drug use, many had taken the protective measures of reducing or eliminating prostitution and IV drug use. When Carlie was asked whether she had been having sex with people for money lately, she responded, "No, I sure haven't . . . ever since they've been talking about AIDS. It kind of scares me and [now] I don't trick and do any of that." Another woman, Francine, described how she had curtailed her drug use and sex life because of the AIDS epidemic:

I am not using needles with anybody whereas maybe in the past I would have. . . . It also makes me aware of not wanting to go out and have sex. . . . I wouldn't have sex with a trick without a rubber anyway. And I would not go around picking men up like some other women [do].

A few women reported leaving their relationships in part due to AIDS risk. Marian had worried about her risk for HIV infection from her husband. She had stayed in the relationship for the sake of their two children. She kept their sexual relationship to a minimum, having sex once every 1 to 2 months. Her statements reflected her fear and attempts to manage that fear: "I think about [AIDS] a lot—if I'm gonna get AIDS from him. That's about it, I just think about it. I don't think I am scared because I don't think he has AIDS. But I'm not sure, so that's why I consider it." A month after her first interview, Marian left her husband for a new relationship with a man who had no drug-use history. The decision seemed to be due to accumulated discontents, with AIDS risk and continued drug use providing the final impetus for leaving.

Feeling Anxious: The Result of Imperfect Strategies

Most women in the study had an overarching sense of risk because their sexual partners were IV drug users, but many were uncertain of the extent of that risk. They had to evaluate the danger secondhand, based on what they knew about their partners' needle practices and sexual contacts. And, despite the efforts they made to protect themselves, the majority remained in relationships in which it was possible to become infected.

Women undertook a variety of measures to reduce their risk for AIDS. Some had curtailed their own IV drug use and sexual contacts, many attempted to influence their partners in safer practices, and the majority had gotten HIV-antibody testing. Still, many women continued to have unprotected sex with men they knew had a history of injecting drugs, and anxiety was the emotional residue of that circumstance. Most knew (at some level of consciousness) that they still could become HIV infected. Sometimes in the course of the brief period of the interview, women seemed to slip into and out of admission of risk for AIDS, or perhaps they conceived of that risk differently depending on the frame of reference. Generally, they knew that women who had sex with IV drug users were at risk, but they described why they would not become infected ("because he tested negative and he's not sharing needles," "because he's careful with his needles," or, for a few, "because we use condoms").

Motivated women devised varied and multiple strategies to reduce the uncertainty regarding their HIV risk and to increase their control over the situation. Despite their efforts, women who continued to have unprotected sex with men who used IV drugs suffered anxiety from lack of knowledge and control over the problem of their HIV risk. For example, Alice's system of denial gave way to acknowledging concern when asked if she was at risk for AIDS in her relationship:

> I would say 99.9 percent no, but there's always that one percent [chance]. He brought home a bag of his dealer's needles, [he said], "just in case we run out [of sterile ones]". . . . So you just never know. I mean he says he's not [sharing], but then there's always that one time that he's going to say . . . "it's OK, I know so and so doesn't have AIDS."

DISCUSSION

Women's incomplete knowledge about their partners' needle practices and lack of control over partners' willingness to use condoms put them in a bind. By the time most women entered the study, they had reduced but not eliminated the activities that put them in danger of acquiring HIV infection. Overall, women saw drug use as the key problem and changes in their partners' drug use as the main solution. Women with IV-drug-use histories themselves had curtailed their drug use and prostitution. Most women in ongoing relationships had attempted to make their partners' drug-use habits safer. Many were instrumental in getting their partners tested. Several had already proposed condom use to their partners; others had avoided the subject because of adverse reactions or their own ambivalence. Avoidance of sex was an option taken by a few women in long-term relationships in which IV drug use continued and condoms were not used.

Public health officials may see condoms as the primary solution to risk, but women sexual partners of IV drug users may not share that view. Women in this study more often conceived of remedies to their risk in terms of some combination of cessation of their partners' risky needle practices, their own avoidance of risk by curtailing IV drug use and sexual contacts, testing of themselves and their partners, and, finally, negotiations with partners over condom use. Testing plus greater needle safety were often preferred to condom use among these couples. Unless the man was known to be HIV infected, condom use was not likely to be seen as imperative, whereas being careful to avoid infection in drug use was often considered important by both members of the couple. Thus changes in needle practices were more likely to be considered as a reasonable demand for the woman to make on her partner.

Negotiations over drug-use practices seemed to be less threatening than negotiations over condoms. Most of the couples had a history of discussing drug use and, however conflictual that topic, negotiations over sex were far more volatile. Proposed changes in drug use could be couched in terms of protecting the man as well as the woman and did not necessarily challenge existing power dynamics. By contrast, a woman's proposal that her partner use condoms raised issues of trust and loyalty, anxieties about sexual performance, and issues of power and control. Especially in couples new to condom use, the introduction of the barrier method often took on symbolic meaning, as in "I need to protect myself from you."

It is not surprising that condom use was not widely adopted among the male partners of these women. The meaning of condom use is linked to deeply rooted norms governing gender roles in heterosexual relationships and to ideologies about sexual identity. Historically, condoms have been used primarily as a form of male protection from sexually transmitted diseases (Himes 1970). Since the nineteenth century in the United States, condoms have been used for contraception primarily in egalitarian marital couples with high motivation to limit the number of children or as a convenient means of avoiding pregnancy in premarital or extramarital sexual encounters (Population Information Program 1982; Degler 1980; Gordon 1976). Research on the effectiveness of condoms for birth control reveals similar patterns, with more successful use among older couples, in longer marriages, among couples highly motivated to prevent pregnancy, and among couples having prior experience with the method (Schirm, Trussell, Menken, and Grady 1982; Laing, Phillips, Zablan, Llorente, and Cabigon 1976; Ryder 1973). When motivation to prevent more births is combined with older age and relatively higher incomes, condom use is extremely effective (Schirm et al. 1982). Cultural and ideological factors influence the participation of both the man and the woman in successful contraception: Hedin-Pourghasemi (1978) found that, among unmarried college men and women, those with the least stereotypical gender attitudes were more likely to have partners who participated in effective contraception. Also suggestive of the need for egalitarian relationships for condom use is the finding that, among single college students, greater emotional involvement and communication about contraception were associated with successful birth control (Maxwell, Sack, Frary, and Keller 1977).

In this study, excluding the couples with men known to be HIV infected, the seven couples who reported consistently using condoms generally fit the above profile. Six were middle class (five white women and one black woman) and four of those six had been using condoms for birth control purposes. Only one woman reported consistently using condoms who did not fit the profile of an effective condom user; she was a former IV drug user who had casual sexual relationships with men who injected drugs. These small numbers do not allow us to generalize, but they suggest that, for those of uncertain HIV risk, sociocultural factors may be the best predictors of condom use, and, more generally, sociocultural factors offer the key to understanding the variations in AIDS risk, conditions and responses.

IMPLICATIONS FOR AIDS
PREVENTION AND RESEARCH

To lower AIDS risk among women, health care providers have attempted to educate and counsel individual women about their possible risks for HIV infection. HIV-antibody testing and counseling have been provided by private and public health facilities. Efforts to reach women at risk outside of clinical settings have been made in several cities, most often as adjuncts to outreach programs for IV drug users. Newspaper and radio coverage of the problem of sexual transmission and pediatric AIDS cases has been helpful in alerting women. Small-scale media efforts have targeted women sexual partners of IV drug users with, for example, video presentations and brochures made available in medical clinics. More widely broadcast media messages have been aimed at gay men or heterosexuals generally and do not adequately address the risk circumstances of women partners of IV drug users, including the important fact that monogamy is not a solution to risk for this group.

Teenagers, IV drug users and their sexual partners, crack addicts, and individuals in poor communities have been dubbed as "hard to reach" populations in the fight against AIDS. However, even "resistant" groups such as IV drug users have been shown to decrease needle sharing and to adopt safer needle-cleaning procedures (Gibson et al. 1989; National Research Council 1989; Sorensen,Batki, Coates, and Gibson 1988). Preventive efforts must reflect the real-life conditions of the groups they speak to and should be carried out by trusted peers, community leaders, and admired public figures. If campaigns against risk practices are to be effective, they must be accompanied by services that can mitigate the immediate risks faced by poor and drug-addicted individuals in their everyday lives. Individuals who inject drugs need sterile needles, drug treatment, health care, job training, and access to additional services. Their women sexual partners need AIDS prevention counseling, anonymous testing, health care, and the other supports that women generally lack—child care, job training and employment opportunities, and affordable housing. Individuals in poor minority communities need most of the above and, additionally, protection from violence in their neighborhoods. Although this is a tall list of needs and additional funds are needed from federal and state governments, existing preventive efforts can be maximized by service providers taking on the additional role of AIDS educators and by prevention programs providing referral and liaison to community services and informal support networks. In addition, grassroots community organizing has the potential to raise awareness, exercise political clout, and provide the support needed to sustain individual and group efforts to avoid HIV-infection risk (Shaw 1988). For example, women in high-risk neighborhoods can become local activists if given access to a copy machine, paper, and safer sex supplies, promoting safety from HIV among their friends and acquaintances.

Media campaigns can affect public consciousness about protection against HIV and, in particular, about condom use. However, there is an intrinsic sexism in campaigns recommending that women get their partners to use condoms. There is a parallel sexism in research aiming to find "ways that women can get their men to wear condoms" (Cohen, Hauer, and Wofsy 1989). There has not been a parallel undercurrent to press for condom use among heterosexual men. Men can be encouraged to use condoms for their own and their sexual partners' safety. Positive encouragement of men and women to be cautious in sexual relationships is likely to be more productive in preventing HIV than pressuring women to exercise control over their partners' use of condoms.

Preventive health models suggest that people are not likely to adopt a preventive health behavior unless they believe they are susceptible to an illness (Siegel and Gibson 1988; Cummings, Becker, and Maile 1980). Women may be more likely to perceive themselves at risk if they have some degree of stability in their lives, such as housing and control over some monetary resources. Addicted, poor, and socially marginal women may be less inclined to consciously register their AIDS risk and are less able to avoid risky situations and behaviors. This does not bode well for the women at highest risk.

More encouraging is the finding that women whose partners currently inject drugs were nearly three times as likely to perceive themselves at risk as women whose partners were no longer injecting (Wermuth,Choi, Ham, Falcone, and Hulley unpublished). It is important to know that women's perceptions of risk are in part based upon the real causes of AIDS risk, in this case, partners' drug injection. These findings, along with the strategies described above, suggest that a subgroup of women are making rational assessments and taking logical steps to reduce their chances of becoming HIV infected.

Very few studies have addressed the interpersonal context of safer sex among heterosexuals. An exception is the study by Magura, Shapiro, Siddiqi, and Lipton (1990), which found that condom use among IV drug users was independently associated with greater personal acceptance of condoms, greater partner receptivity to sexual protection, and recent entry to methadone treatment. In addition, Worth (1989) has pointed out that the ability of women to introduce condom use to their male partners is dependent on relative sexual equality between men and women. Moreover, changes in couples' sex lives require sensitive negotiations. The proposal to adopt condom use affects more than the mechanics of having sex; it may provoke accusations or violence and threaten to end relationships. Additional difficulties arise from the fact that condoms are a male-controlled method over which women can exercise influence but not direct control. And, when faced with partners who refuse to use condoms, economic and emotional dependence may make it difficult for women with children to leave partners who pose an AIDS risk (Mays and Cochran 1988).

A sociological perspective is needed in AIDS behavioral research; factors of social class, interpersonal relationships, gender dynamics, and ethnic/racial class cultures have thus far been neglected. Too often the analysis of AIDS risk and the measurement of behavioral outcomes (e.g., in intervention studies) are reduced to discrete and individual "risk behaviors." This approach often blinds investigators to the cultural and social structural factors that place particular social groups at greater risk for HIV infection. And measurement of risk in heterosexual relationships often does not reflect the asymmetry of control over condom use for men and women. Moreover, because acquiring HIV infection occurs now nearly exclusively in specific behavioral contexts, risk begs to be conceptualized in interpersonal and social contexts. Our studies should examine relationships as a key variable, paying attention to their duration, behavioral norms, level of commitment, emotional and material connectedness, and level of dependency. This applies to drug injectors, heterosexuals, and gay and lesbian couples.

In addressing the needs of women for AIDS prevention efforts, medical treatment, support services, and useful research, there are models that can be adapted. As witnessed among gay men in San Francisco, well-planned and culturally appropriate campaigns can effect dramatic changes (Winkelstein et al. 1988). San Francisco's communities of gay men have demonstrated that grass-roots organizing, mutual support for healthy practices, and group solidarity can slow the spread of HIV and promote the exercise of political clout. Although women sexual partners of IV drug users differ dramatically from this group of largely white, middle-class men, there are useful lessons to be learned for activists and researchers: Solutions must come from within local cultures and resources must be given to agencies and individuals best equipped to influence change. And collaboration between local activists, public health personnel, and researchers is necessary for sound programs and accurate research. This kind of approach holds the greatest promise in reshaping the ideological context of women and AIDS away from that of "vectors of disease" toward that of an empowered group with legitimate needs and demands.

REFERENCES

Ajzen, Icek and Martin Fishbein. 1973. "Attitudinal and Normative Variables as Predictors of Specific Behaviors." *Journal of Personality and Social Psychology* 27:41-57.

Bandura, Albert. 1977. "Self-Efficacy: Toward a Unified Theory of Behavior Change." *Psychological Review* 84:191-215.

Becker, Marshall H. 1974. "The Health Belief Model and Personal Health Behavior." *Health Education Monographs* 2:324-473.

Catania, Joseph A., Susan M. Kegeles, and Thomas J. Coates. 1990. "Towards an Understanding of Risk Behavior: An AIDS Risk Reduction Model (ARRM)." *Health Education Quarterly* 17:53-72.

Centers for Disease Control, U.S. Department of Health and Human Services. 1989a. *HIV/AIDS Surveillance Report* (April). Washington, DC: Author.

Centers for Disease Control, U.S. Department of Health and Human Services. 1989b. *HIV/AIDS Surveillance Report* (July). Washington, DC: Author.

Centers for Disease Control, U.S. Department of Health and Human Services. 1990. *HIV/AIDS Surveillance Report* (January, pp. 1-22). Washington, DC: Author.

Coates, Thomas J., Ronald D. Stall, Joseph A. Catania, and Susan M. Kegeles. 1988. "Behavioral Factors in the Spread of HIV Infection." *AIDS* 2(Suppl. 1):S239-46.

Cocores, James A., A. Carter Pottash, Mark S. Gold, and Norman S. Miller. 1988. "Sexual Dysfunction in Abusers of Cocaine and Alcohol." *Resident and Staff Physician* 34: 57-62.

Cohen, Judith B., Laurie B. Hauer, and Constance B. Wofsy. 1989. "Women and IV Drugs: Parenteral and Heterosexual Transmission of Human Immunodeficiency Virus." *Journal of Drug Issues* 19:39-56.

Collins, Randall. 1974. *Conflict Sociology*. New York: Academic Press.

Cummings, K. Michael, Marshall H. Becker, and Maria C. Maile. 1980. "Bringing the Models Together: An Empirical Approach to Combining Variables Used to Explain Health Actions." *Journal of Behavioral Medicine* 3:123-45.

Degler, Carl. 1980. *At Odds: Women and the Family in America From the Revolution to the Present*. New York: Oxford University Press.

Des Jarlais, Donald C., Samuel Friedman, and David Strug. 1986. "AIDS and Needle Sharing Within the Intravenous Drug Use Subculture." Pp. 111-25 in *The Social Dimensions of AIDS: Methods and Theory,* edited by D. Feldman and T. Johnson. New York: Praeger.

Fullilove, Mindy Thompson, Meryle Weinstein, Robert E. Fullilove III, Eugene J. Crayton, Jr., Richard B. Goodjoin, Benjamin Bowser, and Shirley Gross. Forthcoming. "Race/ Gender Issues in the Sexual Transmission of AIDS." *AIDS Clinical Review.*

Gearing, Frances R. 1974. "Methadone Maintenance Treatment: Five Years Later: Where Are They Now? *American Journal of Public Health* 64(Suppl.):44-50.

Gibson, David R., Laurie Wermuth, Jane Lovelle-Drache, Jennifer Ham, and James Sorenson. 1989. "Brief Counseling to Reduce AIDS Risk in Intravenous Drug Users and Their Sexual Partners: Preliminary Results." *Counseling Psychology Quarterly* 2: 15-19.

Gordon, Linda. 1976. *Woman's Body, Woman's Right: A Social History of Birth Control in America*. New York: Grossman.

Hearst, Norman and Stephen Hulley. 1988. "Preventing the Heterosexual Spread of AIDS: Are We Giving Our Patients the Best Advice?" *Journal of the American Medical Association* 259:2428-32.

Hedin-Pourghasemi, M. 1978. "Sex Role Attitudes and Contraceptive Practices Among Never-Married University Students" (Doctoral dissertation. Tufts University, 1977). *Dissertation Abstracts International* 38:6344A.

Himes, Norman E. 1970. *Medical History of Contraception*. New York: Schocken.

Joseph, Jill G., Susanne B. Montgomery, Ronald C. Kessler, David G. Ostlow, and Camille B. Wortmen. 1988. "Determinants of High-Risk Behavior and Recidivism in Gay Men." Paper presented to the Fourth International Conference on AIDS, Stockholm, June.

Kegeles, Susan M., Nancy E. Adler, and Charles E. Irwin. 1989. "Adolescents and Condoms: Associations of Beliefs With Intentions to Use." *American Journal of Diseases of Children* 143:911-15.

Laing, J. E., J. Phillips, Z. Zablan, R. Llorente, and J. Cabigon. 1976. "The 1974 National Acceptors' Survey." *Population Forum* 2:2-7.

Luker, Kristin. 1975. *Taking Chances: Abortion and the Decision Not to Contracept*. Berkeley: University of California.

Magura, Stephen, Janet L. Shapiro, Qudsia Siddiqi, and Douglas S. Lipton. 1990. "Variables Influencing Condom Use Among Intravenous Drug Users." *American Journal of Public Health* 80:82-84.

Maxwell, J. W., A. R. Sack, P. B. Frary, and J. F. Keller. 1977. "Factors Influencing Contraceptive Behavior of Single College Students." *Journal of Sex and Marital Therapy* 3:265-73.

Mays, Vickie M. and Susan D. Cochran. 1988. "Issues in the Perception of AIDS Risk and Risk Education Activities by Black and Hispanic/Latina Women." *American Psychologist* 43:949-57.

National Research Council Committee on AIDS Research and the Behavioral, Social, and Statistical Sciences. 1989. "Facilitating Change in Health Behaviors." Pp. 259-315 in *AIDS: Sexual Behavior and Intravenous Drug Use,* edited by C. F. Turner, H. G. Miller, and L. E. Moses. Washington, DC: National Academy.

O'Donnell, John A., Karst J. Besteman, and Judith P. Jones. 1967. "Marital History of Narcotics Addicts." *International Journal of the Addictions* 21:21-38.

Padian, Nancy, Linda Marquis, Donald P. Francis, Robert E. Anderson, George W. Rutherford, Paul M. O'Malley, and Warren Winkelstein. 1987. "Male-to-Female Transmission of Human Immunodeficiency Virus." *Journal of the American Medical Association* 256:788-90.

Population Information Program. 1982. "Update on Condoms: Products, Protection, Promotion." *Population Reports* X(5), Series H(6). Baltimore, MD: Johns Hopkins University.

Rosenbaum, Marsha. 1981. "Sex Roles Among Deviants: The Woman Addict." *International Journal of the Addictions* 16:859-77.

Ryder, Norman B. 1973. "Contraceptive Failure in the United States." *Family Planning Perspectives* 5:133-42.

Schirm, Allen L., James Trussell, James Menken, and William R. Grady. 1982. "Contraceptive Failure in the United States: The Impact of Social, Economic and Demographic Factors." *Family Planning Perspectives* 14:68-75.

Shaw, Nancy S. 1988. "Preventing AIDS Among Women: The Role of Community Organizing." *Socialist Review* 100:76-92.

Siegel, Karolynn and William C. Gibson. 1988. "Barriers to the Modification of Sexual Behavior Among Heterosexuals at Risk for Acquired Immunodeficiency Syndrome." *New York State Journal of Medicine,* February, pp. 66-70.

Smetana, Judith G. and Nancy E. Adler. 1979. "Decision-Making Regarding Abortion: A Value × Expectancy Analysis." *Journal of Population* 2:338-57.

Sorensen, James, Steven Batki, Thomas Coates, and David Gibson. 1988. "Methadone Maintenance as AIDS Prevention: Efficacy Three Months Into Treatment." Paper presented to meetings of the American Public Health Association, Boston, November.

Stimmel, Barry, Judith Goldberg, Edith Rotkopf, and Murry Cohen. 1977. "Ability to Remain Abstinent After Methadone Detoxification." *Journal of the American Medical Association* 237:1216-20.

Weinstein, Neil D. 1980. "Unrealistic Optimism About Future Life Events." *Journal of Personality and Social Psychology* 39:806-20.

———. 1982. "Unrealistic Optimism About Susceptibility to Health Problems." *Journal of Behavioral Medicine* 5:441-60.

Wermuth, Laurie, Kyung-Hee Choi, Jennifer Ham, Hsiao-ti Falcone, and Stephen Hulley. Unpublished. "Perceptions of AIDS Risk Among Women Sexual Partners of IV Drug Users."

Wermuth, Laurie and Jennifer Ham. 1989. "The Role of Partner Cooperation in Safer Sex." Paper presented to the meetings of the Society of Behavioral Medicine, San Francisco, March.

Winkelstein, Warren, James Wiley, Nancy Padian, M. Samuel, S. Shiboski, M. Ascher, and J. Levy. 1988. "The San Francisco Men's Health Study: Continued Decline in HIV Seroconversion Rates Among Homosexual/Bisexual Men." *American Journal of Public Health* 78:1472-74.

Worth, Dooley. 1989. "Sexual Decision-Making and AIDS: Why Condom Promotion Among Vulnerable Women Is Likely to Fail." *Studies in Family Planning* 20:297-307.

Zahn, Margaret A. and John C. Ball. 1974. "Patterns and Causes of Drug Addiction Among Puerto Rican Females." *Addictive Diseases* 1:203-13.

5

Sexual Behavior of Male Prostitutes

Rhoda Estep
Dan Waldorf
Toby Marotta

Prior research has established that the three groups most affected by AIDS are male homosexuals, intravenous (IV) drug users, and blood transfusion recipients. However, more current research has identified new groups at risk for contracting AIDS. This study examines one of the groups whose behaviors make them among the most likely to contract the human immunodeficiency virus (HIV)—male prostitutes. All the men studied in this research were prostitutes operating in the San Francisco Bay area. Most of them were also homosexual. In this study, sexual practices were separated into *safe* and *unsafe*, as defined by leading researchers and experts in the field today. Then the major correlates of these safe and unsafe acts were identified.

The research presented here examines these issues in one segment of largely gay men—hustlers and call men. It allowed for a contrast between predominantly middle-class gay males, call men, and a much less often studied group of mainly lower-class gay males, street hustlers. A large proportion of both types of prostitutes are IV drug users. Recently, numerous studies (Friedman et al. 1987; McKusick, Coates, Morin, Pollack, and Hoff 1990; Winkelstein et al. 1987) have concluded that such a characteristic is alarming in light of the finding that gay males are

AUTHORS' NOTE: This research was supported by a grant from the National Institute on Drug Abuse (RO1 DA04535-02).

reducing their risks to a greater extent than IV drug users. One of the major contributions of the research findings presented here concerns whether these two groups of male prostitutes are more closely following the pattern adopted by the bulk of the gay male community or that of IV drug users in risk-taking behavior.

CONTEXT AND LITERATURE REVIEW

The Relationship of Male Homosexuality to Male Prostitution

Most of the early studies of male prostitutes disagreed about the extent of homosexuality among them. For example, one of the first sociological studies (Ross 1959) found that the male prostitutes studied in Chicago claimed to be both homosexuals and prostitutes. In contrast, Reiss (1961), in studying an institutionalized population of predominantly lower-class delinquent male prostitutes, found that virtually none saw himself as homosexual. In fact, he notes incidents of violence after a former client insinuated that the prostitute was a homosexual. When a former customer addressed these prostitutes with a term such as "Sweetie," and they were with other straight males or females, assaults or even murders of customers occurred.

Similarly, although MacNamara (1965) found that sexual preference was primarily homosexual among male prostitutes, Ginsburg (1967) argued that male prostitutes only convert to homosexuality at various times and are primarily heterosexual. Caukins and Coombs (1976) also reported that over 90% of the 41 male prostitutes they studied were not homosexual. In the 1960s and 1970s, however, the gay community grew rapidly and became increasingly political in efforts to establish a gay subculture (Marotta 1981). Subsequent studies on the West Coast (Boyer 1989) have found that the majority of male prostitutes claim to be either homosexual or bisexual.

Rates of Seropositivity Among Male Prostitutes

Given this link between the homosexual subculture and male prostitution, studies on male prostitution in the 1980s began to focus on the men's

HIV status. However, no studies on the issue were published before 1988. One of the first studies on this issue was conducted on Italian prostitutes in Udine, Pordenone, and Treviso (Tirelli et al., 1988). They found that 11% of the 27 prostitutes were seropositive compared with 17% of the 75 homosexual men used as controls. A similar level of seropositivity, 13%, was reported by Dutch researchers after testing 32 male prostitutes working out of brothels in Amsterdam (Coutinho, Van Andel, and Rijsdijk 1988). However, in New York City, many more male prostitutes (53%) tested positive for HIV at the same time (Chiasson et al. 1988). Although the largest sample in these earlier studies was 41, the largest sample of male prostitutes studied prior to the one we report here was conducted on 152 Atlanta street prostitutes (Elifson et al. 1989): 27% were seropositive with the primary risk factors being the number of years they had engaged in prostitution, their sexual orientation, and the average proportion of sexual interchanges involving receptive anal intercourse.

Studies of Gay Men and Safe Sex

Most studies on safe and unsafe sex, however, have been conducted on gay males, who tend to be more middle class than male prostitutes. At least five studies suggest that gay males are increasingly using safe sex practices. Two separate analyses conducted by Martin (1986, 1987) among New York City gays found a decrease in the number of partners, a reduction in anal sex and swallowing semen, combined with a greater use of condoms. Also, in Wisconsin, Golubjatnikov, Pfister, and Tillotson (1983) documented a trend toward fewer sexual partners with a rise in monogamy and celibacy among gay males. Two independent research groups studying San Francisco's gay population identified a similar pattern. McKusick et al. (1990) found there were fewer new sexual partners as well as decreases in anal intercourse among nonmonogamous homosexual males. Similarly, Winkelstein and associates (1987) found a drop in receptive anal sex as well as in the number of partners among those who were seropositive between the beginning of 1984 and the end of 1985.

Nevertheless, the San Francisco cohort study (McKusick et al. 1990) found that almost a fifth of the nonmonogamous subjects were still practicing unprotected anal intercourse in 1988 with higher rates among their monogamous counterparts. They also reported that close to a third had not been tested for the HIV antibody or refused to report their HIV status to the researchers. Thus Stall, Coates, and Hoff (1988) concluded that there are still many opportunities for new HIV infection to occur and, therefore, studies should continue to explore the sexual behavior of gay men.

Previous research on risky behavior provides the context in which to understand the behavior of male prostitutes. First, there is considerable consensus (Bauman and Siegel 1987; Becker and Joseph 1988; Lyman, Asher, and Levy 1986; McCusker et al. 1988) that unprotected anal intercourse is the riskiest sexual behavior for contracting HIV infection. Also, experts agree that anal intercourse is more risky for the receiver than for the insertor. Other practices identified as unsafe include oral-anal contact called rimming, putting hands and/or arms into the rectal cavity known as fisting, and oral-genital sex to the point of ejaculation without the use of a condom (Darrow, Jaffe, and Curran 1983; Darrow et al. 1987; Hennessey and D'Eramo 1986). There are also a few researchers who have questioned the safety of the use of dildos and enemas in sexual activity (Chimel et al. 1987; Hennessey and D'Eramo 1986; Montgomery and Joseph 1988). As a consequence, public health campaigns' major focus has been to try to persuade individuals—in particular, homosexuals, IV drug users, and prostitutes—to abandon anal intercourse or at least use condoms in certain sexual activities.

Correlates of Safe Sex Practices

Numerous factors have been hypothesized to be related to changing sexual practices of certain high-risk groups. The first is knowledge of AIDS. Several studies have established that the greater the knowledge of AIDS, the more likely individuals are to reduce unsafe sexual practices (Carne et al. 1987; Golubjatnikov et al. 1983; Montgomery and Joseph 1988). However, although earlier studies found that increased knowledge about AIDS resulted in risk reduction, recent research has reported a weak association between the two (Ostrow 1989). Becker and Joseph (1988) explain these apparently contradictory effects of knowledge by suggesting a "threshold effect." At first, knowledge creates change, but, at a certain point, additional information does not affect an individual's behavior. For example, among patrons of singles' bars in San Francisco (Stall, Heurtin-Roberts, McKusick, Hoff, and Lang 1990), the heterosexuals' risk-taking behavior was not influenced by their level of knowledge about HIV transmission, and homosexuals were only minimally affected by having such information.

Another factor in risk reduction is number of partners. Several research groups have identified a significant relationship between number of sexual partners and testing positive for HIV (Darrow et al. 1983; Jones et al. 1987; Winkelstein et al. 1987). The third factor possibly influencing the likelihood of contracting AIDS is a person's social class or, as Becker and Joseph (1988) call it, "comparative social advantage." They argue that class may be an intervening variable between knowledge and sexual behavior. The implication for prostitutes perhaps is that the more affluent the prostitute, the more probable that preventive measures like condoms will be used or the most risky behaviors, like anal sex, will be avoided (Rosenberg and Weiner 1988).

In addition, three demographic characteristics have also consistently been identified as significant: age, education, and ethnicity. With respect to age, the evidence suggests that younger gay males are more likely to change sexual patterns than older ones (McKusick et al. 1990). Also, higher educational levels have been found to be associated with safer sexual practices (Coates et al. 1987; Fox, Odaka, Brookmeyer, and Polk 1987; Kaslow et al. 1987). As for ethnicity, nonwhite gay males have been found to be more likely than their white counterparts to change their sexual practices to protect themselves against AIDS (Kaslow et al. 1987).

Finally, a few other dimensions also have been associated with AIDS and the safe sex issue. Several researchers (e.g., Bauman and Siegel 1987) have documented that having an abnormally low level of perceived risk of contracting AIDS results in higher risk taking. McKusick and colleagues' San Francisco cohort study of male homosexuals (1990) reported that being able to visualize someone in the late stages of AIDS—often due to having lost friends to AIDS— was more important than HIV status in reducing risky sexual behavior. Identifying as gay has often been found to be associated with an earlier onset of homosexual activity, thus affording the men more opportunities to contract HIV (Jones et al. 1987). In contrast, another important factor in changing to safer sex is being diagnosed as being HIV positive (Coates et al. 1987; Fox et al. 1987; McCusker et al. 1988). Finally, the combination of engaging in risky sex and being an IV drug user multiplies the risk of being exposed to HIV.

This chapter will identify differences in male street hustlers' and call men's safe and unsafe sex acts. Analysis was undertaken to clarify those factors found to influence sexual practices in these groups. Due to the findings of previous researchers, the emphasis will be placed on the importance of the knowledge of AIDS, the number of sexual partners, IV drug use, and social class in influencing the levels of safe and unsafe sex.

METHODS

Prior to this study, we had considerable information about the world of male prostitutes provided by earlier ethnographic research by one of this chapter's principal researchers. "Hustlers," or male prostitutes who solicit customers in sexual encounters, were found at cruising areas, in gay bars, and at erotic bookstores. They were found to be relatively accessible as well and amenable to being interviewed. Our initial information about "call men," or men who solicit customers over the telephone, via call books, and through advertisements, was more rudimentary; we knew that many of them advertised in specialty newspapers in the area but did not know the range of the different types.

During the process of locating respondents for the study, we formed a typology of male prostitutes that served as a theoretical basis for selecting individuals to be included. The typology is basically an expansion of the original three types suggested by Ross (1959)—bar hustler, street hustler, and call boy. Male prostitutes in San Francisco can be organized into two different general types with various subtypes within each group. The first type, the hustler, is the most visible and the most obvious to the casual observer. Hustlers use face-to-face encounters with potential clients in public and semipublic places. Hustler subgroups are delineated according to erotic styles and sexual identities. They include at least three basic subtypes: trade hustlers, who define themselves as heterosexuals; transvestites, who assume a female identity but define themselves as homosexuals; and gay-identified hustlers, who identify with the larger homosexual community.

The other main type of prostitute consists of call men, who solicit more privately than hustlers. The organization of call men is not based upon erotic styles but on the ways they present themselves to the public and the way they run their business. The three subgroups of call men that we identified in this research were called book men, erotic masseurs, and models or escorts. Call book men obtained customers primarily through the referral method and eventually accumulated a group of regular customers; erotic masseurs obtained customers from massage businesses; and models and escorts obtained customers from advertising.

Based on this ethnographic knowledge, a chain referral sample (Biernacki and Waldorf 1981) was generated, beginning among hustlers at known sites of operation including cruising areas, bars, and erotic bookstores. Call men were located by means of contacts developed by the ethnographer in the study as well as indigenous interviewers and call men known and trusted to provide introductions (Waldorf and Murphy 1990). The respondents consisted of 180 male hustlers and 180 call men living and operating in the San Francisco Bay area. This group of 360 male prostitutes constitutes the largest sample of its kind ever studied to date.

All respondents were interviewed in depth during 1987 and 1988 for 2½ to 4 hours. Interviews consisted of two parts. One was quantitative and structured. The second, a qualitative section, was based on a focused interview guide. The quantitative part included questions on demographic characteristics and on knowledge of AIDS and safe sex, as well as on many other areas discussed in prior research on gay men and AIDS, and it is the basis for this study.

The two groups differed in some ways but not in others. On the average, the hustlers were younger with a median age of 24 years; call men's median age was 30 years. Call men had higher levels of education than the hustlers with median number of years of education 13 years and 11 years, respectively. Both groups were predominantly white. About two thirds of the hustlers and almost three fourths of the call men were Caucasian. All respondents reported having had a fairly religious upbringing, with over half of the hustlers and two thirds of the call men having attended religious services at least once a week while growing up.

Although slightly more than half of the call men's fathers had white-collar jobs, slightly less than half of the hustlers' fathers were so employed. Likewise, slightly more of the hustlers' than the call men's fathers held blue-collar jobs. With respect to mothers' occupations, few differences were found, with one exception. Although over a third of the call men's mothers had been housewives, this was true of less than a fourth of the hustlers' mothers. Overall, then, the occupational status of their parents indicated that the call men were from more affluent families. As has been found in previous studies on parents' occupation and sexual activity (Forste and Heaton 1988), the higher the parents' social status, the more likely their offspring are to engage in responsible sex. Based upon these demographic findings, we hypothesized that hustlers would be more likely to engage in more risk-taking behavior than call men.

Also noteworthy was the finding that over two thirds of the call men were gay identified, compared with less than half of the hustlers. Additionally, almost a quarter of the hustlers described themselves as being transvestites. Because of these differences in levels of gay identification among the two main types of prostitutes studied here, it seemed important to ask additional questions about their partners and the sexual activities in which they were engaged. We, therefore, asked about eight types of sex partners, both male and female, in each of the four following categories: intimates, friends or acquaintances, anonymous nonpaying partners, and customers. Over nine tenths of both groups had had a male client in the previous week. Because of the very low level of reported contact with female customers found among these men, contacts with male customers became the main focus of our analysis.

FINDINGS

The eight acts this study identified as "safe sex" encompass mutual masturbation, body rubbing or frottage, hugging and kissing, and prophylactically protected anal or oral-genital contact (see Table 5.1). Both groups reported that they had engaged in the highest number of safe sex acts with customers compared with other partners in the last week. Both hustlers and call men also were found to have almost identical levels of safe sex acts in the previous week, with 4.4 acts and 4.5 acts, respectively. Among the other partners of the hustlers, the mean number of safe sex acts was lowest with anonymous nonpaying partners (.6), higher with friends or acquaintances (.7), and higher still with intimates (1.2). Overall, call men had slightly higher levels of safe sex acts with all categories of partners than did the hustlers. However, the order paralleled that of the hustlers. The call men reported an average of 1.6 safe sex acts with intimates, 1.5 with friends or acquaintances, and 1.2 with anonymous nonpaying partners. The fact that the highest level of safe sex occurred with clients can be attributed to the finding that these men had more customers than any other type of partner. Thus more partners in the client category resulted in a larger number of safe sex acts with customers.

The nine acts identified as unsafe here included anal intercourse without a condom, fisting, rimming, and oral-genital contact without a condom, with or without ejaculation (see Table 5.1). Except with customers, call men reported a higher mean number of unsafe sex acts with all other partners than did hustlers. With respect to customers, however, hustlers reported an average of 1.9 unsafe sex acts, whereas call men averaged 1.4 in the last week. With other partners, hustlers averaged .5 unsafe sex acts with intimates, .4 with friends or acquaintances, and .3 with anonymous nonpaying customers. After clients, call men were most likely to be involved in unsafe sex with intimates (.7), followed by friends or acquaintances (.6), and least often with anonymous nonpaying partners (.5).

Table 5.1 Safe and Unsafe Sex Practiced by Male Prostitutes with Other Males During the Past Week

	Hustlers				Call Men			
	Intimates %	Friends/ Acquaintances %	Anonymous Partners %	Clients %	Intimates %	Friends/ Acquaintances %	Anonymous Partners %	Clients %
Safe sex acts:								
mutual masturbation, respondent to another	76.0	53.1	68.0	81.4	82.8	88.2	87.8	86.6
mutual masturbation, respondent himself with others	61.2	54.8	68.0	75.0	75.9	92.2	92.7	81.7
frottage (body rubbing)	65.3	54.8	68.0	62.6	72.4	70.6	70.7	75.0
frottage to the point of orgasm	40.8	38.7	48.0	49.4	43.1	54.0	51.2	52.4
hugging and kissing	90.0	77.4	72.0	59.9	93.1	90.2	85.4	71.3
receptive anal intercourse with a condom	42.0	45.2	32.0	31.4	38.6	31.4	37.5	27.4
insertive anal intercourse with a condom	32.0	29.0	36.0	49.1	49.1	60.8	52.5	51.2
oral-genital sex with a condom	40.0	58.1	24.0	49.1	31.6	36.0	42.5	45.7
Unsafe sex acts:								
receptive anal intercourse without a condom	32.0	32.3	32.0	21.6	12.3	21.6	10.0	5.5
insertive anal intercourse without a condom	26.0	22.6	28.0	18.1	15.8	11.8	10.0	8.5
passive fisting (respondent received)	0.0	6.5	0.0	4.1	5.3	7.8	7.5	3.0
active fisting (partner received)	2.0	6.5	0.0	4.7	7.0	15.7	12.5	11.0
oral-anal stimulation (rimming) (respondent received)	14.0	41.9	32.0	21.8	36.8	31.4	32.5	27.6
oral-anal stimulation (rimming) (partner received)	10.0	29.0	24.0	8.7	26.3	22.0	25.0	11.7
oral-genital sex without a condom	54.0	64.5	60.0	64.1	80.7	76.0	87.5	57.9
ejaculation into partner's mouth without a condom	32.0	32.3	36.0	37.1	24.6	20.0	25.0	23.8
ejaculation into respondent's mouth without a condom	24.0	19.4	15.8	17.1	15.8	14.0	12.5	7.4
Number of respondents cases	(50)	(32)	(25)	(172)	(58)	(51)	(41)	(164)

NOTE: Percentages are based on the number of cases at the bottom of each column. Cases represent the number of respondents who admitted to having sexual contact during the previous week.

The most glaring discrepancy between hustlers and call men was the fact that four times as many hustlers as call men reported engaging in unprotected receptive anal intercourse during the previous week. Hustlers also were substantially more likely to report having unprotected anal intercourse than were the call men. Call men engaged in fisting (partner received), for example, among friends, acquaintances, and anonymous partners more than the hustlers did. Also, call men conducted oral-genital sex without a condom more often than did the hustlers. These differences once again reflect the fact that more call men than hustlers were gay identified and largely reserved certain intimate acts for intimates or other gay-identified partners. Also, these variations may illustrate the class difference between the two groups of prostitutes, illustrating the more desperate situation of the hustler.

To more fully understand the various important dimensions of these men's life-styles in regard to their safe and unsafe practices with customers, we compare relative levels of key variables of sex-related activities between call men and hustlers (see Table 5.2). A major similarity between the hustlers and call men was the high level of general and specific AIDS knowledge they possessed. Call men averaged correct responses on 38 of the 45 questions whereas hustlers were not quite as knowledgeable (36.5) on overall AIDS knowledge; however, both indicated a very high level of knowledge about AIDS. Regarding knowledge of safe sex, call men averaged 7 correct answers to the 8 questions and hustlers were basically as aware as the call men, averaging 6.9 correct responses. Also, in both groups, about two thirds had been tested for HIV. Overall, more differences than similarities appeared between the two types of prostitutes. Hustlers provided services to almost twice as many customers during the previous week as did call men (8.6 versus 4.9). However, call men were more likely than hustlers to have had sex with an AIDS, ARC, or HIV-positive male in the past; known someone having AIDS, ARC, or testing positive for HIV; believed they had been exposed to the AIDS virus; known someone who had died of AIDS; or tested positive for HIV themselves. Finally, 23% of the call men and 11% of the street hustlers self-reported being HIV positive.

In bivariate analyses, overall knowledge of AIDS, number of clients in the past week, age, whether they used drugs intravenously, and whether they had known someone who died from AIDS were significantly related to safe and unsafe sex for both groups. Numerous other factors were found to have only a negligible relationship with safe or unsafe sex acts for these

Table 5.2 Selected Independent Variables Hypothesized to Affect
Male Prostitutes' Safe Sex Practices

	Hustlers %	Call Men %
Those tested for HIV	68.9	62.8
Those having had sex with an AIDS victim	10.0	41.1
Those having had sex with someone with ARC	10.0	37.8
Those having had sex with someone testing positive for HIV	13.3	43.3
Those knowing someone having ARC or AIDS	65.9	81.1
Those knowing someone testing positive for HIV	65.9	79.4
Those who believe they have been exposed to the AIDS virus	24.2	33.8
Those knowing someone who has died of AIDS	56.4	73.3
Those testing positive for HIV	10.6	22.9
Those having injected a drug	61.5	38.1
Those being gay identified	44.4	67.8
Number of cases	(180)	(180)

male prostitutes. These variables included ethnicity, educational level, fathers' and mothers' occupational status, religiosity while growing up, knowledge of people with a positive HIV, ARC, or AIDS status, and having had sexual partners with a positive HIV, ARC, or AIDS status.

The independent behavior variables chosen to be entered into the multiple regression were based on previous analyses both here and elsewhere. The three factors most strongly supported by the literature as influencing safe or unsafe sexual practices were knowledge of AIDS, knowledge of safe sex, and the number of clients in the previous week. Four other factors we hypothesized to be relevant included whether or not the prostitute was an IV drug user, whether he felt he had been exposed to the AIDS virus, whether he had known someone who died of AIDS, and his age. All of the above were entered into regression equations to explain safe and unsafe sex.

Although it would have been desirable to include each prostitute's HIV status in the regression analysis as well, we decided against its inclusion for several reasons. We were only able to obtain the HIV status on three fifths of those interviewed because the remaining two fifths, for the most part, had never been tested. Because multiple regression eliminates all cases with missing data on the variables entered, the number of cases would have been considerably reduced if we had included HIV status as an independent variable.

A "forced entry" regression analysis in SPSSX was employed to determine the relative effect of the seven independent variables (see Table 5.3). Dummy variables were used for being an IV drug user, being exposed to HIV, and having known someone who died of AIDS. The most important predictor of both safe and unsafe sex acts found here was the number of customers encountered during the past week. The two other independent variables found to significantly explain sexual practices among call men were whether the prostitute had known someone who died from AIDS and whether he had ever injected drugs. Both for the overall sample and, particularly, for call men, those having known someone who died from AIDS were more likely to refrain from unsafe sex. In contrast, those who were IV drug users were more likely to engage in unsafe sex. Knowledge, both in general and more specifically, on safe sex failed to reach significance in the regression. Multicollinearity between these two items was ruled out as an explanation because this failure to reach significance held true even when the knowledge items were separately added to the regression equations. Although the beta weights associated with age and exposure to HIV failed to reach significance, the direction of the correlations was as predicted; that is, younger prostitutes engaged in more safe sex acts; older call men, in more unsafe sex; and those hustlers who felt they had been exposed to the AIDS virus were more likely to engage in both safe and unsafe sexual activities.

Using Cronbach's alpha (Cronbach 1951), reliability for the scale measuring the safe sex items was .71 whereas reliability was .65 for the unsafe sex scale. For example, among the safe sex items, the highest intercorrelation was between frottage and continuing that effort until orgasm occurred ($r = .65$). None of the interim correlations in the unsafe sex scale was above .50. Knowledge about AIDS and its transmission is highly subjective and produces much disagreement. It is extremely probable that future research efforts will be able to improve existing reliability coefficients. Reliability for safe and unsafe sex scales will increase when researchers begin to report the number and types of acts done in a single encounter by male prostitutes and the relative riskiness of each sexual activity. Such information can be used to enhance reliability by assigning weights to the items that correspond to the probability that HIV will be transmitted by that action.

Table 5.3 A Multiple Regression Analysis of Safe and Unsafe Sex Acts

Independent Variables	Entire Sample		Hustlers		Call Men	
	Safe Sex[a] (Beta Weights)	Unsafe Sex (Beta Weights)	Safe Sex (Beta Weights)	Unsafe Sex (Beta Weights)	Safe Sex (Beta Weights)	Unsafe Sex (Beta Weights)
Overall knowledge of AIDS	.06	.09	.02	.08	.02	.12
Knowledge of safe sex	.07	.10	.04	.07	.07	.12
Number of clients in previous week	.20**	.26**	.16	.24*	.35***	.24*
Intravenous drug user	.00	.15*	-.03	.09	.04	.19*
Exposure to the AIDS virus	.05	.08	.17	.16	-.03	.02
Knowing someone who died of AIDS	.02	-.16*	-.04	-.14	.05	-.20*
Age (in years)	-.13	.03	-.14	-.01	-.13	.15
R^2	.07*	.14***	.07	.13*	.16*	.15*

a. Indexes representing safe and unsafe sex are simply an addition of any act within each category in which the prostitute engaged during the past week. Thus, the indexes do not reflect the frequency with which the acts occurred and so avoid possible multicollinearity with the number of clients serviced in the previous week.
$*p < .05; **p < .01; ***p < .001.$

DISCUSSION

The average number of safe sex acts for both call men and hustlers with their clients was between four and five separate activities per week. For both groups, over twice as many safe sex as unsafe sex acts occurred with male customers. Hustlers were found to average almost two unsafe sex acts with customers per week, compared with one and a half for call men.

Possible explanations for the differences varied by the type of prostitute. For call men, the number of clients was by far the most significant variable in predicting the amount of safe and unsafe sex. Greater levels of general knowledge of AIDS increased the number of safe sex acts with customers for the call men. It also enhanced the probability that more unsafe sex acts were involved in the transactions as well. Among call men, knowledge about AIDS had the potential effect of increasing the number of *both safe* and *unsafe* sex acts. This apparently inexplicable and unexpected finding has also been found by other researchers on this topic (Becker and Joseph 1988; Ostrow 1989). On the other hand, the relationship between hustlers and their clients was significantly affected by neither general knowledge of AIDS nor specific knowledge of safe sex and AIDS.

The fact that the number of clients served was the single, most significant variable points to the importance of the social context in which these two distinctive levels of male prostitutes were operating. Compared with the call men, the hustlers catered to roughly twice as many clients per week. Because of the smaller number of regular clients, the call men were more likely than the hustlers to know the HIV status of their sexual partners. Although the hustlers believed they were less at risk for contracting AIDS, this was possibly due to the anonymous, transitory nature of their encounters with customers. Hustlers tended to congregate in areas of high drug use and to dwell within poor neighborhoods, often in cheap hotels. The relative social advantage of the call men allowed them to live in a more affluent social environment, which gave them the ability to choose their customers and the acts they performed more cautiously.

In conclusion, then, the different types of male prostitutes have been discovered to be extremely important in the sexual risk taking that occurs. Call men are extremely sophisticated and, even when involved in technically "unsafe" sex such as anal intercourse, often insist upon withdrawal before ejaculation in an effort to protect themselves against AIDS. In contrast, hustlers constitute a more diverse population of males. The ones whose style could be characterized as transvestite think of themselves as more like a female prostitute and use condoms more often. (This development has been made possible in part by the outreach efforts of organizations like COYOTE [Call Off Your Old Tired Ethics] and CAL-PEP [California Prostitute Education Project, for female prostitutes].) Likewise, those hustlers with female intimates may be more cautious in their sexual activities with customers than the gay-identified hustlers.

The final group of hustlers, which constituted half of this category and were exclusively gay identified, were the most likely of all the male prostitute groups to engage in unprotected anal intercourse. Additionally, they reported frequently using amphetamines intravenously to get emotionally ready for their work, which reduced their inhibitions and is thought to have led to more unsafe sex. As a consequence of the gay-identified hustlers' life-style, they were more economically deprived and thus were driven to take more risks, which made them increase their probability of contracting HIV.

With respect to AIDS prevention, various approaches need to be shaped to accommodate the male prostitutes described above. The gay-identified call men could be approached through peers and gatherings within the gay subculture. Their relatively high level of education means written information regarding AIDS in gay newspapers could have a substantial impact on their behavior as well. The importance of communicating with the entire gay subculture should not be underestimated in future AIDS prevention efforts. Lower-class hustlers would probably be the toughest to convince of the importance of protecting themselves from AIDS. Street outreach workers or drop-in centers where free bleach or syringes and condoms are available would probably be the most efficient method of reaching this type of hustler.

Additionally, prevention efforts must begin to target the heterosexual males who are frequently customers of these male prostitutes. One of the most graphic reminders of this fact was revealed by a call man who reported that one of his customers had a car equipped with two infant car seats. Hence, we contend that male prostitution is definitely a way HIV is spreading. AIDS will remain a threat to everyone until all segments of society are educated regarding its transmission and an insistence on sexual honesty about the activities of all sexual partners becomes normative.

REFERENCES

Bauman, Laurie J. and Karolyn Siegel. 1987. "Misperception Among Gay Men of the Risk for AIDS Associated With Their Sexual Behavior." *Journal of Applied Social Psychology* 17:329-50.

Becker, Marshall H. and Jill Joseph. 1988. "AIDS and Behavioral Change to Reduce Risk: A Review." *American Journal of Public Health* 78:394-410.

Biernacki, Patrick and Dan Waldorf. 1981. "Snowball Sampling: Problems and Techniques of Chain Referral Sampling." *Sociological Methods and Research* 10:141-63.

Boyer, Debra. 1989. "Male Prostitution and Homosexual Identity." *Journal of Homosexuality* 17:151-84.

Carne, C. A., A. M. Johnson, F. Pearce, A. Smith, R. S. Tedder, I. V. D. Weller, C. Lovely, A. Hawkins, P. Williams, and M. W. Adler. 1987. "Prevalence of Antibodies to Human Immunodeficiency Virus, Gonorrhea Rates, and Changed Sexual Behavior in Homosexual Men in London." *Lancet* 1:656-58.

Caukins, Silvan E. and Neil R. Coombs. 1976. "The Psychodynamics of Male Prostitution." *American Journal of Psychotherapy* 30:441-51.

Chiasson, M. A., A. R. Lifson, R. L. Stoneburner, W. Ewing, D. Hildebrandt, and H. W. Jaffe. 1988. "HIV Seroprevalence in Male and Female Prostitutes in New York City." In *Proceedings of the IV International Conference on AIDS*. Stockholm, June.

Chimel, Joan S., Roger Detels, Richard Kaslow, Mark Van Ruden, Laurence A. Kingsley, Ron Brookmeyer, and the Multicenter AIDS Cohort Study Group. 1987. "Factors Associated With Prevalent Human Immunodeficiency Virus (HIV) Infection in the Multicenter AIDS Cohort Study." *American Journal of Epidemiology* 126:568-78.

Coates, Thomas J., Ron Stall, Jeffrey S. Mandel, Alicia Boccellari, James L. Sorer en, Edward F. Morales, Stephen Morin, James A. Wiley, and Leon McKusick. 1987. "AIDS: A Psychosocial Research Agenda." *Annals of Behavioral Medicine* 9:21-28.

Coutinho, R. A., R. L. M. Van Andel, and T. J. Rijsdijk. 1988. "Role of Male Prostitutes in Spread of Sexually Transmitted Diseases and Human Immunodeficiency Virus." *Genitourinary Medicine* 64:207-8.

Cronbach, Lee J. 1951. "Coefficient Alpha and the Internal Structure of Tests." *Psychometrika* 16:297-334.

Darrow, William W., Dean F. Echenberg, Harold W. Jaffe, Paul M. O'Malley, Robert A. Byers, James Getchell, and James W. Curran. 1987. "Risk Factors for Human Immunodeficiency Virus (HIV) Infections in Homosexual Men." *American Journal of Public Health* 77:479-83.

Darrow, William W., Harold W. Jaffe, and James W. Curran. 1983. "Passive Anal Intercourse as a Risk Factor for AIDS in Homosexual Men." *Lancet* 2:160.

Elifson, Kirk W., Jackie Boles, Mike Sweat, William W. Darrow, William Elsea, and R. Michael Green. 1989. "Seroprevalence of Human Immunodeficiency Virus Among Male Prostitutes." *New England Journal of Medicine,* 321:832-33.

Forste, Renata T. and Tim B. Heaton. 1988. "Initiation of Sexual Activity Among Female Adolescents." *Youth and Society* 19:250-68.

Fox, Robin, Nancy J. Odaka, Ron Brookmeyer, and B. Frank Polk. 1987. "Effect of HIV Antibody Disclosure on Subsequent Sexual Activity in Homosexual Men." *AIDS* 1:241-46.

Friedman, Samuel R., Don C. Des Jarlais, Jo L. Sotheran, Jonathan Garber, Henry Cohen, and Donald Smith. 1987. "AIDS and Self-Organization Among Intravenous Drug Users." *International Journal of the Addictions* 22:201-9.

Ginsburg, Kenneth. 1967. "The Meat Rack: A Study of the Male Homosexual Prostitute." *Journal of Psychotherapy* 21:170-85.

Golubjatnikov, R., J. Pfister, and T. Tillotson. 1983. "Homosexual Promiscuity and the Fear of AIDS." *Lancet* 2:681.

Hennessey, N. Patrick and James E. D' Eramo. 1986. "Update: AIDS Related Complex (ARC)." *Medical Aspects of Human Sexuality* 20:22-35.

Jones, Clifton, Betty Waskin, Brigid Gerey, Betty J. Skipper, Harry F. Hull, and Gregory Mertz. 1987. "Persistence of High-Risk Sexual Activity Among Homosexual Men in an Area of Low Incidence of the Acquired Immunodeficiency Syndrome." *Sexually Transmitted Diseases* 14:79-82.

Kaslow, Richard A., David G. Ostrow, Robert Detels, John Phair, Frank Polk, and Charles M. Rinaldo for the Multicenter AIDS Cohort Study. 1987. "The Multicenter AIDS Cohort Study: Rationale, Organization, and Selected Characteristics of the Participants." *American Journal of Epidemiology* 126:310-18.

Lyman, David, Michael Asher, and Jay A. Levy. 1986. "Minimal Risk of Transmission of AIDS-Associated Retrovirus Infection by Oral-Genital Contact." *Journal of the American Medical Association* 255:1701-3.

MacNamara, Donald E. J. 1965. "Male Prostitution in an American City: A Pathological or Socioeconomic Phenomenon." *American Journal of Orthopsychiatry* 35:204.

Marotta, Toby. 1981. *The Politics of Homosexuality.* Boston: Houghton Mifflin.

Martin, John L. 1986. "AIDS Risk Reduction Recommendations and Sexual Behavior Patterns Among Gay Men: A Multifactorial Categorical Approach to Assessing Change." *Health Education Quarterly* 13:347-58.

———. 1987. "The Impact of AIDS on Gay Male Sexual Behavior Patterns in New York City." *American Journal of Public Health* 77:578-81.

McCusker, Jane, Anne M. Stoddard, Kenneth H. Mayer, Jamie Zapka, Charles Morrison, and Scott P. Saltzman. 1988. "Effects of HIV Antibody Test Knowledge on Subsequent Sexual Behaviors in a Cohort of Homosexually Active Men." *American Journal of Public Health* 78:462-67.

McKusick, Leon, Thomas J. Coates, Stephen F. Morin, Lance Pollack, and Colleen Hoff. 1990. "Longitudinal Predictors of Reductions in Unprotected Anal Intercourse Among Gay Men in San Francisco: The AIDS Behavioral Research Project." *American Journal of Public Health* 80:978-83.

Montgomery, Suzanne B. and Jill G. Joseph. 1988. "Behavioral Change in Homosexual Men at Risk for AIDS: Intervention and Policy Implications." *New England Journal of Public Policy* 4:323-34.

Ostrow, David G. 1989. "AIDS Prevention Through Effective Education." *Daedalus* 118: 229-54.

Reiss, Albert J., Jr. 1961. "The Social Integration of Queers and Peers." *Social Problems* 9:102-20.

Rosenberg, Michael J. and Jodie M. Weiner. 1988. "Prostitutes and AIDS: A Health Department Priority?" *American Journal of Public Health* 78:418-23.

Ross, H. Laurence. 1959. "The 'Hustler' in Chicago." *Journal of Student Research* 1:13-19.

Stall, Ron D., Thomas J. Coates, and Colleen Hoff. 1988. "Behavioral Risk Reduction for HIV Infection Among Gay and Bisexual Men." *American Psychologist* 43:878-85.

Stall, Ron, Suzanne Heurtin-Roberts, Leon McKusick, Colleen Hoff, and Sylvia Wanner Lang. 1990. "Sexual Risk for HIV Transmission Among Singles-Bar Patrons in San Francisco." *Medical Anthropology Quarterly* 4:115-28.

Tirelli, Umberto, Emanuela Vaccher, Pierluigi Bullian, Silvana Saracchini, Domenico Errante, Vittorina Zagonel, and Diego Serraino. 1988. "HIV-1 Seroprevalence in Male Prostitutes in Northeast Italy." *Journal of Acquired Immune Deficiency Syndromes* 1:414-17.

Waldorf, Dan and Sheigla Murphy. 1990. "Intravenous Drug Use and Syringe-Sharing Practices of Call Men and Hustlers." Pp. 109-31 in *AIDS, Drugs, and Prostitution*, edited by Martin A. Plant. New York: Tavistock/Routledge.

Winkelstein, Warren, Jr., Michael Samuel, Nancy S. Padian, James A. Wiley, William Lang, Robert E. Anderson, and Jay Levy. 1987. "The San Francisco Men's Health Study III: Reduction in Human Immunodeficiency Virus Transmission in Homosexual/Bisexual Men, 1982-1986." *American Journal of Public Health* 76:685-89.

Part III
The Social Context
of Treatment and Policy

6

Organizing Drug Users Against AIDS

Samuel R. Friedman
Meryl Sufian
Richard Curtis
Alan Neaigus
Don C. Des Jarlais

Other than gay men, intravenous drug users (IVDUs) account for more AIDS cases than any other group in the United States. Sexual HIV transmission from IVDUs, and perinatal transmission from IV-drug-using women or the infected female sexual partners of IV-drug-using men, have been the source of most heterosexual and perinatal transmission AIDS cases in the United States. The epidemic among IVDUs initially was concentrated in the New York metropolitan area but is increasingly national and international in scope. Thousands of IVDUs also have been infected in other countries, including Spain, Italy, France, and Thailand (Des Jarlais et al. 1989; Des Jarlais and Friedman 1988a). In studies as early as 1984, more than half the IVDUs in New York City reported having attempted to reduce their risks, and many studies have found that interventions to increase risk reduction among IVDUs lead to positive behavioral change. Nonetheless, considerable risk taking continues and

AUTHORS' NOTE: The research in this chapter was supported by National Institute on Drug Abuse Grant No. DA05283 and by a grant for AIDS Outreach Project Research from the New York State Division of Substance Abuse Services. The views expressed in this chapter do not necessarily reflect the positions of the granting agencies or of the institutions in which the authors are employed.

new infection also continues to occur, although the prevalence of infection among IVDUs seems to have leveled off in some parts of New York City, in Stockholm, and in Innsbruck (Des Jarlais et al. 1989). Thus new ways need to be developed to increase the extent of AIDS risk reduction among IVDUs. This chapter describes such an intervention.

Gays have organized to deal with AIDS in many cities. They have spoken up for their interests and thus helped shape governmental and other policy responses, have set up care for the sick, and have provoked a dialogue among gays over appropriate ways to reduce HIV transmission. These activities have led to considerable declines in new infection among gays with ties to organized gay subcultures (Friedman, Des Jarlais et al. 1987; Coutinho, van Grievson, and Moss 1989; Stall, Coates, and Hoff 1988).

IVDUs have not organized so readily. Unlike gay men, they have not undergone a (drug-injectors') liberation movement or established political influence in major cities. In the absence of such a base, they have lacked organizational resources to establish AIDS organizations. They have also faced severe repression. (The theoretical basis for this analysis of IVDUs and organizing, and its relationships to social movement theory, has previously been described in Friedman and Casriel 1988.)

The Netherlands are a partial exception to this picture. IVDUs there organized drug users' unions (*junkiebonden*) in the early 1980s to get more tolerance and respect as well as to win better treatment by government and medical institutions. They began needle exchange programs to reduce hepatitis B risks (these were later expanded by the government in response to the AIDS threat) and have actively worked for risk reduction in IVDUs through word of mouth, leaflets, pamphlets, and working with local user groups to make videos as an educational tool. Their ability to organize was facilitated by repression of drug use being less severe in the Netherlands than in many other countries (de Jong 1986; Friedman, de Jong, and Des Jarlais 1988). Although the degree to which authorities in the Netherlands allow drug sales and use is often distorted in the media, and sellers of hard drugs often face long prison terms, drug policy has much more of a public health approach than in the United States. Thus Dutch authorities have been willing to accept the fact that drug users have a right to political representation, and much of their policy has focused on harm reduction rather than repression (Buning, van Brussel, and van Santen 1988).

Although current users have not organized in the United States, New York City ex-users and sympathetic health professionals set up ADAPT (the Association for Drug Abuse Prevention and Treatment). After encountering considerable difficulty in defining its role and finding capable leadership, ADAPT became an important actor in AIDS-related issues by 1987. It has tried to educate IVDUs about AIDS and to provide a voice for the interests of IVDUs in AIDS policy discussions. As of the beginning of 1990, it had about a dozen outreach workers on its staff and was engaged in a project to provide training in AIDS interventions in a number of cities in the United States. It also has been a major proponent of needle exchanges as a tactic in the fight against AIDS, which has led to some controversy between it and other minority-led organizations in New York City (Des Jarlais, Casriel, Stephenson, and Friedman forthcoming.)

Both the junkiebonden and ex-users' groups like ADAPT have found the lack of available leaders to be problematic. This has been especially severe for the junkiebonden. Although they have had a few effective leaders in particular cities and on a national level, these leaders have had great difficulty in establishing a core of secondary leadership and likewise have had trouble finding replacements for themselves when they have personally become less active in the organizations. Typical patterns are that promising new leaders either become so involved in their addiction that they have no time for organizing or get imprisoned on drug-related charges.

REASONS FOR ORGANIZING IVDUs IN THE CONTEXT OF AIDS

Although drug users' organizations can serve many other interests as well, here we will consider their roles in combating AIDS. Drug users' organizations have three major AIDS-related functions. First, they can provide a political voice concerning health care and public policy. ADAPT, for example, is a vocal proponent of needle exchanges and of increased drug-abuse treatment availability, and the junkiebonden have been active participants on government committees to set AIDS policy. Second, drug users' organizations also can set up buddy systems and other direct services for the sick. This was done by ADAPT for people with AIDS in New York jails. Finally, and perhaps most important, drug users' organizations can work within drug-using subcultures to convince other users to reduce their risks and to support each other in risk reduction.

Here, we present a preliminary report on an attempt by Narcotic and Drug Research, Inc. (NDRI), and ADAPT (as a subcontractor to NDRI) to set up organizations of IVDUs who are still injecting to battle for risk reduction.[1] This project was set up in the belief that current users are more a part of the IV drug subculture than are ex-users and also in the belief that change is more easily won if it can be fought for by insiders rather than by outsiders. Because, however, IVDUs were not themselves spontaneously organizing against AIDS, we attempted the somewhat contradictory task of organizing from the outside to work for change inside the IVDU subculture.

This discussion focuses first on process data; these data reflect ethnographic observations and interviews as well as the experience of NDRI staff as participants in the process. As such, it has a significant participant observation component, and the views expressed here may have been shaped by our active involvement in and commitment to the project. The chapter then turns to a brief presentation of preliminary data comparing behavior change among two groups: IVDUs in the neighborhood where the organizing project took place and IVDUs who received AIDS education from a standard outreach project.

Analysis of the Organizing Process

At the beginning of the project, it was not at all clear that outside organizing of IVDUs could successfully occur. Based on ethnographic observations of the organizing efforts in the project, it now seems that organizing can indeed occur, and (as discussed below) it leads to risk reduction. On the other hand, many questions remain for further research—including some that are fundamental to strategic decision making about whether or not organizing should be promulgated as a national initiative.

We found that it is possible to hold recurrent meetings of IVDUs, that it is possible to involve IVDUs on an ongoing basis in assisting in many concrete tasks (such as filling and distributing bleach bottles), that some IVDUs are willing to spend considerable time in a location where a project is taking place, and that potential leaders can be located and involved in the process. Although we developed useful experience in these areas, we have not yet succeeded in creating a core of self-consciously involved indigenous drug-injecting organizers or in determining how self-sustaining and expansionistic organizations could be set up. As is discussed below, our difficulties in these areas largely arose because organizing was not carried to stages in which IVDUs would have initiative that was at all independent of staff control.

The organizing project was originally conceived of as having several stages. These were first, winning trust and acceptance from local drug injectors; second, getting them to use the storefront as a place to hang out for informal discussion and, relatedly, to attend weekly meetings in our storefront to discuss risk reduction, organizing strategies, tactics, and events; third, systematic leadership identification and development; fourth, truly indigenous leadership coordinating and initiating collective activity to try to change the IV-drug-user subculture in ways that would promote risk reduction; and, fifth, expansion and replication of drug-user organizations against AIDS under the leadership of active drug injectors. Significant progress was made in the first two of these stages, and some evidence exists to suggest that the third and fourth could be done with serious prospects for success. This evidence is presented below in terms of the different stages.

(1) Winning trust and acceptance. Outside organizing is always difficult, whether the people being organized are residents of poor communities, are workers, or are drug injectors. One key obstacle is developing initial trust. This was accomplished over a 6-month period through the use of ex-user organizers to provide intensive AIDS education outreach, including the distribution of bleach and condoms, and to provide assistance in getting users medical assistance and other services.

(2) Establishing the storefront as a hangout and holding weekly meetings. Once a storefront was opened near a major local "copping" area (a location where drugs are sold in the street), it became a drop-in center for local drug injectors, particularly those women who engaged in prostitution at a local "stroll." Many of these women were in their twenties or late teens and deeply engaged both in smoking crack and in injecting heroin, cocaine, or heroin and cocaine mixed in a "speedball."

Weekly group meetings of women who are both IVDUs and prostitutes had begun in July 1988, 5 months after the project entered the field. Attendance averaged 11, with a range between 6 and 20. The women's group was clearly the most successful IVDU group meeting held at the storefront. Discussions at women's group meetings covered a wide variety of topics including drug use, antibody testing, safer sex with customers and with other sex partners, safety in dealing with customers, streetwise safety practices, how to cope with HIV infection, and many other health issues.

A men's group, which held meetings somewhat sporadically, was less successful than the women's group, perhaps because it focused primarily on therapy rather than organizing. Regular meetings did not begin until July 1989. Attendance averaged 8, and ranged between 3 and 18. Discussions at men's group meetings covered many of the same topics that were discussed at women's group meetings; however, they differed in that the approach taken by group leaders (staff members) in the men's group was much more oriented toward individual problem solving than group action.

(3) Systematically identifying and developing leadership. During the first phase of the project, some efforts were made at identifying and working with potential leaders. For example, one way the staff built trust was to bring food and a table to set it out at a local copping area/hangout once a week. They observed which of the drug users took the initiative in helping them set up and clean up and in keeping order during distribution. Similarly, they observed which drug injectors took initiative and responsibility by helping to distribute bleach to others.

Leadership development, on the other hand, was subordinated to other concerns and interests of top leadership at the subcontractor organization. They redirected ideas that had been seen as a way to develop leadership into one-shot publicity events for their organization that did not further leadership development among the IVDUs. One example was a plan to work with identified leaders to organize a collective building cleanup at an abandoned building where many users lived and injected drugs. Refuse, such as used syringes, bloody cotton, and other contaminated material, formed a thick layer in almost all areas of the building, and the residents wanted to clean it up. An organizing tactic such as the cleanup can build self-esteem and collective identity among all participants and can give the users who help plan and direct it considerable leadership training. The top leadership of the subcontracting organization, however, let their need for organizational recognition interfere with the organizing. They one day decided to bring a reporter the next day. Staff were simply told to be sure that enough users were on hand to clean up the building. Enough groundwork had been laid for the media event to occur successfully, but very little leadership development took place. Further, in spite of line staff desires, no follow-up cleanups in this building or others took place, which prevented the initial cleanup from becoming the basis for subsequent organizing successes.

This event exemplifies three dynamics that are important for future attempts to organize IVDUs: First, the value of media coverage to sponsoring organizations can disrupt the organizing effort (see also the experience in the Minneapolis/St. Paul project as described in Carlson and Needle 1989). Second, ex-user organizations like ADAPT put other institutional interests above those of building organizations of current users (see below). Third, and most important, it shows that organizing is a *process* rather than an *event* and that it involves an interconnected chain of activities and events that build upon each other to create the social skills, interconnections, and roles that constitute organizations.

Similarly, leadership identification occurred through the group meetings in the storefront, and indeed officers were elected by the women's group (which chose the name "Women in Progress" for itself). However, this did not lead to leadership development and organization building but to the development of dependency for four prominent reasons: First, group meetings tended to attract the most dysfunctional users in the neighborhood. (To some extent, this was a product of a deliberate joint decision to locate the project in a neighborhood with a large number of the worst-off IVDUs in the city.) Those who were recruited for group meetings were extremely needy: homeless, without family or other significant social support networks, jobless, outside the circuit of public welfare agencies, and in poor health. They were typically attracted to the project by the offer of a warm place to sit, free food during the meetings, and other similar assistance rather than because of any special interest in organizing themselves against AIDS. Although there is no doubt that IVDUs such as these are—and should be—a target of AIDS intervention projects, their high degree of dysfunction meant that they may have been less promising as an initial target of organizing than other IVDUs who were more functional. This parallels the experience of the junkiebonden in the Netherlands, who have found that few of their effective leaders are at the dysfunctional end of addiction (de Jong 1986).

Second, the initial organizing staff resigned at the beginning of 1989 due to discontent with obstacles put in the way of their attempts to organize. Replacement staff were given minimal or no training in how to organize. Thus they conducted group meetings using methods and techniques that were familiar to them as a result of their experiences as clients and counselors in therapeutic communities.

Their approach tended to be confrontational rather than supportive, atomizing rather than cohesiveness building, judgmental rather than understanding, and oriented toward individual therapy and problem solving rather than group action. Two examples of what happened at group meetings will help make this clear:

In a women's meeting, a female staff member admonished the entire group: "I'm not going to stop talking to you about changing your life. I'm going to keep after you!" Then, as if to emphasize her point and show them that she was intent upon confronting them, she singled out for stinging criticism a woman who had been going through a rough period in the last several weeks. She told T that, because of her untreated disease (not related to HIV), she was going to "end up dead in the streets." During the "lecture" T. kept quiet. There was very little she could say to rebut those predictions, but she certainly didn't like being singled out in front of the group.

The men's group was also the site of both moralizing at, and confrontations with, members. During one meeting, a staff member asked the participants to show them how a condom was used. He provided them with a broomstick to demonstrate the technique. After each participant had done so, he told several members who had come late for the meeting (and thus missed his demonstration of how it should be done) that they had used the condom improperly. The staff member then proceeded, in front of the group, to make fun of these "men" who "couldn't even use a condom the right way." Of course, these men did not appreciate being told that they were less than "real" men, and did not attend many meetings after that embarrassment.

Third, top subcontractor officials sidetracked efforts to build users' leadership skills and conscious collective self-organization. One startling example of this is that potential leaders who had attended many group meetings and were interviewed by the process ethnographer were not even aware that the project aimed to foster user self-organization. Another is that a health fair for the neighborhood, originally conceived of by organizing staff and group attenders as a group-building collective effort, became a staff-conducted project. A desire to avoid offending neighborhood sentiment led the top subcontractor leadership to relegate users to the sidelines and minimize their involvement in planning the event. Field staff were discouraged from involving the users they were supposed to be organizing.

Fourth, some potential leaders entered drug abuse treatment or other social services (such as resident shelters). This had positive effects upon them as individuals but also meant that they no longer were part of the local drug scene and thus did not develop as leaders for drug-user organization. This dynamic, which we had anticipated from before the start of the project, restricted organizational growth less than would otherwise have occurred because relatively little organizing was happening.

(4) Coordinating and initiating by active drug injectors. As discussed above, top subcontractor leadership, and sometimes the organizing staff themselves, prevented the systematic development or even the spontaneous flowering of users' own initiatives and collective coordination of activities. Nonetheless, we frequently observed cases in which IVDUs suggested activities for the group and others in which they wanted to take responsibility for carrying out group projects (as in the health fair, where users volunteered to take responsibility for balloons and food but were shunted aside). The level of initiative that did occur suggests that much more can be accomplished if initiative is encouraged.

(5) Expanding and replicating drug-user organizations. The organizing in this project never developed to the point at which expansion and replication could become a realistic possibility. It is worth noting that the Minneapolis-St. Paul project did find that a small user organization they established was able to encourage another group to form with only minimal aid from the Twin Cities project staff (Carlson and Needle 1989).

Lessons About Staffing and Subcontracting

The statistical analyses presented below indicate that the organizing project was moderately successful in encouraging bleach use and, indeed, that it had more of an impact than did the outreach project (which educated about bleach but only rarely distributed it). Ethnographic evidence also supports the finding that bleach use increased. Nonetheless, success in institutionalizing bleach use among IVDUs was constrained in several ways. Review of ethnographic field notes indicates that bleach was not made available on a regular basis in IV-drug-user circles: Supplying shooting galleries with gallon containers of bleach was done only sporadically, staff often did not carry bleach with them while conducting outreach, and the organizing storefront (run by the subcontractor) went through several periods when bleach was not available for weeks at a time. It is significant to note that, even with irregularity of supply, bleach use among IVDUs did indeed increase.

Another source of difficulty in the project's attempt to institutionalize bleach use among active IVDUs was the extreme reluctance of field staff (all of whom were ex-IVDUs) to spend long periods of time in shooting-up locations, whether to observe, organize, or exhort IVDUs actually to use bleach. Current practice in most cities uses ex-IVDUs as the most knowledgeable people with respect to IVDU subcultures. This, however, need not imply willingness to reenter that subculture. Indeed, our observations strongly suggest that ex-IVDUs are in some ways inappropriate for this task because many of them have invested several years of their lives in rejecting this life-style. Thus asking them to reenter this subculture empathically grates against deep feelings they have come to have during their recovery from their own addictions. Given their obvious revulsion for this subculture, it was not surprising that the project's ethnographer did not record any instances when staff members spent more than ten minutes in any location where active shooting-up was taking place. To some extent, this may have been a product of the personnel policies and "official doctrine" (Selznick 1959) of the subcontracting organization, and we know there are individual exceptions among outreach workers in other cities. Nonetheless, we conclude from this that organizing teams in such projects should be composed of a mixture of ex-users and of never-users with organizing skills and experience.

We also suggest that ex-user community organizations or drug treatment agencies may not be appropriate groups to attempt to organize IVDUs. They are subject to intellectual and emotional pressures to see IVDUs as "clients" who need treatment, and this seems to conflict with organizing them to take collective action on their own initiative. Similarly, the success of an organization of IVDUs could pose a threat to their own organizational interests, whether in terms of undermining commitments to views that drug users are too enslaved by their addictions to lead useful lives or by raising the prospect that the users' organization may critique the "parent" organization. Evidence from the Minneapolis-St. Paul project that drug-abuse treatment agencies became hostile to their organizing project supports this argument (Carlson and Needle 1989). Having said this, we do not have any definitive conclusions about what organizations might be most appropriate to conduct such outside organizing. Research organizations might have the ability, but some might also be subject to pressures leading them to withdraw from such projects. Community-based AIDS organizations, or perhaps activist groups (such as ACT UP or the European Movement for the Normalization of Drug Policy, which has been involved in sponsoring trips by ex-junkiebond activists to try to initiate self-organization by users in different cities) might be appropriate agencies.

QUESTIONNAIRE DATA

Methods

Organizing as a public health intervention is unlike many forms of intervention in that it attempts to enlist those members of the target population who have become involved in the project as active agents in changing the risk behaviors of other people who are at risk. This has important methodological implications. Project success should be evaluated in terms of its impact on all the IVDUs in the neighborhood, not only on those who came into direct contact with the project. Thus we interviewed IVDUs who live or inject drugs in the neighborhood. The data for these subjects were compared with data on a comparison group of IVDUs. Comparison group members had all taken part in a "standard" outreach project in which ex-addict educators talked with them about the risks of AIDS and tried to recruit them for HIV-antibody testing. This comparison is an extremely conservative test: It compares standard outreach subjects (all of whom received some individual intervention) with subjects from the neighborhood in which the organizing occurred, regardless of whether they had had contact with the project. Furthermore, the sample from the organizing project may have been diluted somewhat by IVDUs from outside the neighborhood who came to get money, because subjects who were interviewed received $15 for their time and effort both at intake and at follow-up.

Subjects were interviewed about AIDS-related behaviors, beliefs, knowledge, and medical history. A follow-up interview was then administered at a 6-month interval. The instruments used for the data reported here were the AIDS Initial Assessment and the AIDS Follow-up Assessment. They are being used by over 50 projects around the United States. (Data on the extent of subjects' direct involvement in the project and the extent to which they had tried to get other IVDUs to reduce their risks were also collected but are not reported here.) In keeping with the definitions of the national research design, no subjects had been in drug-abuse treatment within the 30 days prior to intake, and all had injected drugs within the previous 6 months.

The following are preliminary data about behavior change. Between the start of the project and May 31, 1989—the cutoff date for these analyses—intake interviews were conducted with 529 organizing and 446 standard outreach subjects. Of these, 259 (49%) organizing and 223 (50%) outreach subjects have been reinterviewed, so far, at a median of

196 days later. Subjects who have and have not yet been followed up were similar in gender and project (organizing versus outreach) and in intake values of dependent variables. Subjects were significantly more likely to have been reinterviewed if they were older (mean age 34.3 among subjects followed up versus 32.8 for those not), were black (42% of those followed up, 32% of those not), were Latino (44% versus 54%), had a conventional place to live (66% versus 60%), or used shooting galleries less (18% of injections in the six months prior to intake by those followed up versus 24% among those who were not.)

These data are preliminary in several ways. Perhaps most important, the study is not yet over, so that the subjects reported here are those who both took part in the first 60% of the project and also were among the first subjects to be tracked down for follow-up. Thus it is possible that later analyses will produce different results if these initial subjects turn out to have been a biased sample. Also, analyses to ascertain whether these results differ for persons of different age, gender, race, or other antecedent variables have just begun.

Results

Data on incidence per month of drug injection and of vaginal or anal sex without a condom are shown in Table 6.1. Repeated measure t tests are used to determine whether significant change occurred within each project. Analysis of variance with repeated measures was used to determine whether behavior changed significantly between outreach and organizing (where the probability is that of the interaction between project and time). Table 6.2 presents data on the percentage of subjects who were taking particular steps to reduce their risks. McNemar's chi-square for paired observations is used to test whether changes in these proportions are significant.

Subjects from the Williamsburg area (where the organizing project took place) report considerable reduction in risk. They reduced total drug injections from a mean of almost six per day to four per day; this included significant declines in injection frequencies of heroin, cocaine, and speedball. There also were significant increases in the proportion of organizing subjects who always used new needles and then disposed of them without using them a second time, always used bleach, and always used condoms.

Subjects who received individual AIDS education (and perhaps antibody counseling and testing) also reduced their drug injection frequency,

Table 6.1 Comparison of Change in Frequency of Drug Injection and Unprotected Sex of Outreach and Organizing Subjects

Dependent Variable Project	Means at Interview 1	Means at Interview 2	Difference of Means	p of Mean Difference Within Program	p for Difference by Program <
Drug injections/month:					
organizing	171	120	–51	.0001	.10
outreach	137	66	–71	.0001	
Cocaine injections/month:					
organizing	39	31	–8	.0111	.11
outreach	37	20	–16	.0001	
Heroin injections/month:					
organizing	65	48	–17	.0001	.0014
outreach	57	23	–34	.0001	
Speedball injections/month:					
organizing	67	41	–26	.0001	.57
outreach	44	21	–23	.0001	
Vaginal/anal sex without condoms/month:					
organizing	9	11	+2	.29	.08
outreach	16	13	–3	.17	

and the proportions of such subjects who always use new needles and who always use condoms increased significantly. Their bleach use did not significantly increase. The mean monthly frequency of sex without a condom did not decline significantly in either group (in spite of the fact that a minority of subjects in each project did begin to use condoms all the time).

The analysis of differences in outcomes between the two projects is extremely preliminary, because follow-up is incomplete and multivariate analysis has barely begun. These preliminary analyses indicate a significantly greater decline in mean heroin injection frequency among outreach subjects, which may be a result of the fact that organizing subjects were injecting more at intake (and thus may have had more trouble reducing their addictions to both cocaine and heroin) but that organizing subjects had a significantly greater probability of adopting bleach use for all injections ($p < .05$) and condom use whenever they had sex ($p < .05$).

Table 6.2 Percentages Attempting Risk Reduction Measures at
Intake and Follow-Up (outreach and organizing subjects)

Variable	Intake %	Follow-Up %	p (McNemar's chi-square)
Always use new needle:			
organizing	7	20	.0005
outreach	9	24	.0005
Always use new needle and then always dispose of it after one use:			
organizing	4	11	.01
outreach	6	13	.10
Always use bleach to decontaminate syringe:			
organizing	7	19	.005
outreach	4	8	ns
Always use condoms during sex:			
organizing	23	34	.03
outreach	12	21	.03

CONCLUSIONS

There are two kinds of conclusions that can be drawn from the findings
in this chapter. On the basis of project experience, we can conclude that
the results of having "outside organizers" attempt to organize IVDUs
against AIDS are by no means chimerical. Considerable progress was
made in this project in spite of the difficulties that arose in implementing
it. Furthermore, as discussed above, a number of specific practical lessons
were learned about how to implement such organizing in the future.

Second, analysis of the survey data indicates the project led to considerable risk reduction. Indeed, these preliminary analyses indicate that the
organizing project initiated greater "harm minimization" through the use
of bleach and condoms among the IVDUs in the neighborhood than did
individual outreach. These findings suggest that the organizing approach
is worth pursuing.

An Unanswered Question

It has been 9 years since AIDS was discovered. Considerable risk
reduction has occurred among IVDUs, but it remains partial and incon-

sistent. The resources allocated to preventing HIV transmission among IVDUs remain extremely limited. In New York City, there are fewer than 100 outreach workers for an estimated 200,000 IVDUs. It seems unlikely, furthermore, that any qualitative increase in the ratio of outreach workers to IVDUs will occur.

The strategy of organizing IVDUs offers the possibility of surmounting this resource imbalance and of creating subcultural change that may lead to and maintain consistent risk reduction. The success of the strategy is by no means guaranteed; indeed, full success requires several problematic sets of events to occur. IVDUs organizations have to be established; they have to become self-sustaining; and they have to develop a momentum that leads to their spreading and organizing new IVDU groups throughout New York City (and, perhaps, beyond it). In this chapter, we have by no means demonstrated that this is possible. What we have done is more modest: We have shown that even a limited organizing project can lead to considerable risk reduction; we have discussed some of the difficulties inherent in organizing and suggested some ways in which these difficulties might be overcome; and we have shown that it is not absurd to think in terms of IVDUs' organizations as a strategy in the battle against AIDS. Given the alternatives, we suggest that further efforts to organize IVDUs against AIDS are both necessary and worthwhile.

NOTE

1. NDRI is a nonprofit organization that conducts research and training related to drug use, its causes, and its effects. It also has an AIDS Outreach Project that provides drug injectors and their sexual partners with HIV education and referrals to a variety of social and medical services.

REFERENCES

Buning, Ernst, Giel van Brussel, and Gerrit van Santen. 1988. "Amsterdam's Drug Policy and Its Implications for Controlling Needle Sharing." Pp. 59-74 in *Needle Sharing Among Intravenous Drug Abusers: National and International Perspectives,* edited by R. Battjes and R. Pickens. NIDA Research Monograph 80. Washington, DC: Government Printing Office.

Carlson, Gregory and Richard Needle. 1989. "Sponsoring Addict Self-Organization (Addicts Against AIDS): A Case Study." Presented to the First Annual National AIDS Demonstration Research Conference, Rockville, MD.

Coutinho, Roel, Godfried van Grievson, and Andrew Moss. 1989. "Effects of Preventive Efforts Among Homosexual Men." *AIDS* 3(Suppl. 1):S53-S56.

de Jong, Wouter. 1986. "De sociale Beweging van Opiatengebruikers in Nederland." Doctoraal-scriiptie Sociologie, Erasmus Universiteit, Rotterdam.

Des Jarlais, Don, Cathy Casriel, Bruce Stephenson, and Samuel Friedman. Forthcoming. "Expectations of Racial Prejudice in AIDS Research and Prevention Programs in the United States." *Drugs and Society.* 5:1-7.

Des Jarlais, Don and Samuel Friedman. 1988a. "HIV and Intravenous Drug Use." *AIDS* 2 (Suppl. 1):S65-S69.

———. 1988b. "The Psychology of Preventing AIDS Among Intravenous Drug Users: A Social Learning Conceptualization." *American Psychologist* 43:865-70.

Des Jarlais, Don, Samuel Friedman, David Novick, Jo Sotheran, Pauline Thomas, Stanley Yancovitz, Donna Mildvan, John Weber, Mary Jeanne Kreek, Robert Maslansky, Thomas Spira, and Michael Marmor. 1989. "HIV-1 Infection Among Intravenous Drug Users in Manhattan From 1977 Through 1987." *Journal of the American Medical Association* 261:1008-12.

Friedman, Samuel and Cathy Casriel. 1988. "Drug Users' Organizations and AIDS Policy." *AIDS and Public Policy* 3:30-36.

Friedman, Samuel, Wouter de Jong, and Don Des Jarlais. 1988. "Problems and Dynamics of Organizing Intravenous Drug Users for AIDS Prevention." *Health Education Research* 3:49-57.

Friedman, Samuel, Wouter de Jong, Don Des Jarlais, Charles Kaplan, and Douglas Goldsmith. 1987. "Drug Users Organizations and AIDS Prevention: Differences in Structure and Strategy." Presented to the Third International Conference on AIDS. June.

Friedman, Samuel, Don Des Jarlais, Jo Sotheran, Jody Garber, Henry Cohen, and Donald Smith. 1987. "AIDS and Self-Organization Among Intravenous Drug Users." *International Journal of the Addictions* 22:201-19.

Friedman, Samuel, Jo Sotheran, Abu Abdul-Quader, Beny Primm, Don Des Jarlais, Paula Kleinman, Mauge Conrad, Douglas Goldsmith, Wafaa El-Sadr, and Robert Maslansky. 1987. "The AIDS Epidemic Among Blacks and Hispanics." *Milbank Quarterly* 65 (Suppl. 2):455-99.

Nadelmann, Ethan A. 1989. "Drug Prohibition in the United States: Costs, Consequences, and Alternatives." *Science* 245:939-47.

Selznick, Philip. 1959. *TVA and the Grass Roots.* New York: Harper.

Stall, Ron, Thomas Coates, and Colleen Hoff. 1988. "Behavioral Risk Reduction for HIV Infection Among Gay and Bisexual Men." *American Psychologist* 43:878-85.

7

From Burying to Caring: Family AIDS Support Groups

Barbara G. Sosnowitz
David R. Kovacs

The continuing spread of HIV and the attendant increase in diagnosed cases of AIDS in the United States pose an increasing challenge to the formal and informal mechanisms of care for diagnosed individuals. Although state and local governments are beginning to address the professional care needs of persons with AIDS (PWAs) from a medical and psychosocial perspective, similar resources and energies have yet to be expended on the disease in a larger social context involving the non-professional caregivers who are a part of the PWAs' lives. This group includes partners/spouses, friends, parents, siblings, and relatives as well as designated others. These caregivers, by choice or by accident, share the vagaries experienced by all caregivers of the chronically and terminally ill. They, like all caregivers, must take on additional roles and regimes to cope with the adversity of illness and the necessities of maintaining life (Cogswell 1976; Strauss and Glaser 1975). In addition, caregivers of PWAs have emotional stresses that appear to be exclusive to them. Due to the condemnation of some of the behaviors that lead to the HIV infection, these stresses often revolve around secrecy and the need to manage information given to other family members, neighbors, and employers. The fear of contagion also exposes them to rejection from traditional sources of help such as emergency and medical services.

Mental health literature is replete with research indicating that social support can reduce anxiety and distress during times of stress. Recent studies (Kasl 1983; Taylor, Falke, Shopaw, and Lichtman 1986) have increasingly recognized that family support, combined with social factors, can influence an individual's response to illness. Anderson and Bury (1988) suggest that contributions of family and other informal carers are the main ingredient of community care—a fact that itself has become the foundation of health and social services for people with chronic illness. However, there has been little recognition of the consequences of an individual's illness on the family or on the person charged with ongoing care.

The notion that people dealing with a stressful situation will derive comfort and support by comparing and contrasting personal feelings and emotions with others in like circumstances is an underlying factor in the development of peer support groups. Early examples of self-help groups in the United States include Alcoholics Anonymous and Synanon (Hurwitz 1976). The growth and popularity of self-help support groups in the United States continue unabated. As many as 6 million Americans are using self-help support groups to cope with chronic conditions (Taylor et al. 1986). Myriad human issues and stressors currently are being examined within this structure. Issues range from agoraphobia to cancer to women's concerns.

As the number of PWAs increases each year, the number of people in need of social service increases. Traditional organizations providing health and social services have not expanded to meet this demand (Appleby and Sosnowitz 1988). They have been slow to react to the epidemic and are just now starting to educate themselves about the disease. The involvement of traditional social service agencies with AIDS services in Connecticut, for example, first appeared to have monetary motivation, the result of increased federal dollars. However, it now appears to be more of a formality, one used to maintain professional credibility. These agencies continue to be remiss in developing specific services for PWAs. Programs are being developed along traditional patterns, which do not meet the needs specific to this disease, including the entire spectrum of psychosocial, medical, and political support. It is not surprising then, to see the development of self-help and support groups to deal with the various aspects of AIDS ignored by the professional community.

There are several factors that appear to contribute to the necessity of peer support. One is the current sociopolitical climate in the United States.

Eight years of Reagan conservatism have left a deep imprint on human services provision from the local to federal levels (Appleby and Sosnowitz 1988). The core philosophy is that the local community, guided by concerned individuals, is best able to determine local needs and solutions to problems. This leaves the community and the family with greater responsibility for its members (Sosnowitz and Appleby 1988). One result of this policy, as applied to AIDS, has been the formation of local AIDS projects and task forces to meet the immediate and ongoing needs of infected individuals and their caretakers.

A second factor affecting the provision of service to PWAs is the concept of the individual as responsible for contracting the disease. There has been a general tendency by health providers to "blame the victim," suggesting patients did not follow regimes or seek medical care soon enough (Crawford 1986; Knowles 1986), and in periods of cost cutting, persons with an illness are accused of not paying attention to public health warnings, relying too heavily on medical services, and not using their own resources sufficiently (Crawford 1986). Some of the practices of homosexual men and IV-drug-using persons may result in the spread of HIV. These practices are seen as deviant or morally reprehensible by the majority of Americans (Levitt and Klassen 1979). This has resulted in a tendency to cast the PWA as deserving or having brought about his or her fate (Patton 1985). This willingness to ascribe guilt or blame has become complicated by the spread of AIDS to hemophiliac and pediatric populations. In response to this, the popular press has employed the term "innocent victim" in referring to these two newer risk groups. By comparison, gays and IV drug users would be labeled "guilty" or perhaps deserving victims. This continued moral enshroudment of the AIDS epidemic poses problems for all those associated with the disease, including the nonprofessional caregiver (Sosnowitz and Appleby 1988).

A recent study (Kelly, St. Lawrence, Smith, Hood, and Cook 1987) of the attitudes of physicians toward PWAs bears out the pervasiveness of negative attitudes toward PWAs. Randomly selected physicians in three cities were asked to evaluate one of four narratives that described a patient with AIDS or leukemia. Patients were identified as being either homosexual or heterosexual. These physicians were then asked to complete a set of attitude measures regarding the narrative they had read. "Physicians considered the AIDS patient to be more responsible for his illness, more deserving of what has happened to him, . . . to be less deserving of sympathy and understanding, more dangerous to others, and more deserving of quarantine" (Kelly et al. 1987, p. 790). Clearly, the implications of findings such as these are a cause for concern. More research needs to be done regarding the veracity and incidence of such attitudes in the professional caregiving community. The immediate implications for PWAs and their informal caregivers are serious. Traditional avenues of support for dealing with a terminal disease have not been as readily available to those affected by AIDS. Much of the emotional support of PWAs and their loved ones has come from support services provided by local AIDS projects. One such service has been the implementation of support groups for caregivers of PWAs. This chapter will use anecdotal material to discuss issues raised and experienced in a support group designed to address the needs of nonprofessional caregivers of PWAs. By summer 1990, the group had been in existence for over 3 years.

AIDS Project/Hartford (AP/H), from whose clients the information for this chapter was derived, was founded in March 1985. As with many other AIDS projects across the nation, AP/H was initially the response of the local gay community to a situation receiving scant response and support from traditional agencies (Appleby and Sosnowitz 1988). As AP/H has grown, its volunteer base has broadened to include nonprofessional and professional volunteers working to provide the many services needed by the AIDS-infected community.

The establishment of direct services for PWAs in the form of "buddies" and support groups quickly brought volunteers into direct contact with the caregivers of our primary clients. The majority of these caregivers (parents, spouses/lovers, friends, and siblings) as well as their infected loved ones were experiencing emotional trauma. Anecdotal reports of "buddies"—volunteers who were asked to "just listen" to some of the problems experienced by caregivers as they tried to make sense of the disease in a social context of fear and secrecy—plus the experiences of the authors—whose function at that time was intake evaluation—pointed up the need for an ongoing support mechanism for caregivers of PWAs.

At this time, there are four major groups of individuals affected by AIDS: gay/bisexual men, IV drug users and their partners, hemophiliacs and others receiving infected blood products, and the children of HIV-infected mothers. The informal network of caregivers responding to each of these groups shared certain issues but also experienced other issues exclusive to the risk group with which their loved one was affiliated.

The first support group for caregivers of PWAs in Connecticut was formed in May 1987. The ideas in this chapter are based upon our experience as cofacilitators of that group as well as on the observations and experiences of the group members themselves over a period of 2 years. As participant observers concerned with providing care, we tried to pay attention to events as they occurred in each caregiver's life. "Evaluation research that traces particular outcomes to particular conditions and events inherent in the program provides a realistic base for redesign as well as providing guidelines for the development of new programs" (Cogswell 1968, p. 440). When it was time for us to terminate our participation, we collaborated with the group to write this chapter. As part of the disengagement process, we wrote our report, and the group of caregivers critiqued it.

AIDS has spread among groups of people who often are considered to be functioning outside traditional societal expectations. Thus, at times, their caregivers, those emotionally close to the PWAs, are not included in traditional definitions of family (Schneider 1984). The *family caregiver,* as related to AIDS, includes and goes beyond the roles traditionally associated with the term. Spouses may be of the same or opposite sex. Partners may be functioning in relationships without the benefit of, or in defiance of, traditional societal sanctions. Siblings and other relatives may be actively involved with and accepting of the PWA life-style or actively condemning and rejecting of the infected individual's behaviors and partners. All may, however, end up being responsible for the daily care of a PWA. As Michael Bury (1988, p. 92) suggests, "There is no guarantee that significant others will respond in a wholly predictable or supportive manner;" with illnesses, "the contingencies of family life and the expectations that members have of relationships are all put under threat."

One result of the stigma associated with AIDS is that primary caregivers may also be close friends as well as "designated caregivers," that is, volunteer buddies from a local AIDS project. Additionally, in many pediatric cases, where the biological mother may already have died of AIDS, the parent-caregivers can be foster care participants, if the child is lucky, or nurses and volunteers available on a hospital pediatrics unit. Experience with this group over time has led to the identification of a number of emotional reactions that we suspect are commonly experienced by most caregivers of PWAs.

PREMATURE BURIAL

Although each PWA and his or her caregiver responds to the disease of AIDS within his or her own coping patterns, we noted a tendency on the part of new caregivers to be in a deep stage of grief—as if the PWA were very near death. This reaction on the part of the caregiver proved to be based more in emotionality than founded on a factual prognosis. At the same time, other members seemed to be in a panic, terrified by the illness and what it would mean to them personally. A fear of loss of the loved one and of their close relationship and an impending upheaval of their lives was almost more than they could bear. They were "prematurely burying" their loved one. One young man related: "We made our wills, got things in order, took a special vacation, you know, all the things we'd been putting off. And then things kinda went on hold. It's like I was waiting for him to die."

This feeling of overwhelming loss and emotionally burying the loved one was commonly experienced by all the caregivers we worked with in the group. Robinson (1988) noted a similar pattern in studying families who had a member with multiple sclerosis. He found that the impact of a diagnosis was generally more negative for the families of persons with multiple sclerosis than it was for the patients themselves.

This period of seeing the PWA, often recently diagnosed, as almost dead frequently lasted several months. Although seasoned members of the group began to point out the fact of premature burial to new ones, this realization was typically brought about by interaction between the PWA and the caregiver. Most of the caregivers were forced to deal with their grief in an abrupt manner. One father described how he was forced to face this fact: "I was sitting with my son. I must have looked really depressed or something, because he all of a sudden said 'Hey, dad! C'mon. I'm not dead yet. Don't bury me till I am.'" The young man quoted here had just recovered from his fifth bout of PCP (pneumocystis carinii pneumonia), demonstrating the increasing chronicity of AIDS.

DENIAL

Denial, the second reaction we noted in caregivers, was manifested in a variety of ways and seemed to be a complete reversal of their original reactions. Talk in the group was often centered on plans for the future, when he or she "gets better." This feeling was often shared with the PWA and, together with the caregiver, he or she would spend large sums of money purchasing automobiles, VCRs, and other pleasurable items. It was as if the caregiver and the PWA had a sense they would receive bad news in the future but it had not arrived yet. Pinder (1988, p. 69) offers an explanation when she writes,

> Balancing is, of course, an activity in which we are all engaged. Where the chronically ill differ is in the nature of the considerations that are traded off. Most people predicate their lives on the notion of an orderly, predictable and inherently stable world. Plans are made in the reasonably confident expectation of their materializing. This is essentially a survival device, protecting us from experiencing the world as intolerably anarchic.

This period of denial that we witnessed appeared to allow time for the caregiver to come to grips with the fact that AIDS can be a chronic disease. This has become a major change in the epidemic as medical advances increase the life expectancy of those afflicted with the disease. People are now "living with AIDS," putting additional strains on the providers of care.

Spouses of PWAs, whether gay or straight, may tend to use the denial mechanism for different purposes. Because AIDS is a sexually transmitted disease, partners of PWAs are faced with the possibility that they too may be infected. Of seven partners in the caregiver group, only one had been tested for HIV after learning of his loved one's diagnosis. When questioned about this, the most common response from individuals was that they needed all of their strength to take care of their loved ones. Most viewed the possibility of their own infection as an added stress with which they did not want to cope. Although half of the group are typically partners of PWAs, group discussion rarely touches upon the physical health of any group member.

ANGER

Although the caregiver of a PWA does face grief reactions common to others dealing with different chronic illnesses, there are reactions to AIDS that appear to be fairly exclusive to this disease. When caregivers cease to deny their situation, they often display a great deal of anger in group meetings. This anger is often intense, is directed at a wide variety of individuals and institutions, and is partially a direct result of the intense stigma that surrounds AIDS.

Social isolation is perhaps one of the most salient features of AIDS. It is imposed not only by society but by the caregivers themselves. This can be summarized by a woman whose husband, a hemophiliac, had received infected blood products: "There's just no one I can yell at! I don't dare tell people at work what the real problem is, and I can't take it out on [my husband]. This is the only place I feel like I can really let go." Sharing anger and frustration in the group setting is a frequent event. Individuals functioning as caregivers to PWAs soon find themselves on an emotional roller coaster. The natural course of the disease involves frequent periods of relapse and remission of symptoms, progress as new drugs or therapies are tried, seeming periods of arrest and new vigor, followed by new opportunistic infections, which create a feeling of frustration with the PWA. Another caregiver, a young man, relates a feeling common to caregivers in the group who feel guilty about their anger:

> I'm feeling angry at him because our whole relationship is changing. I have to be the strong one all the time. It used to be we could share problems. I could turn to him for support. Now I don't feel like I can load him down with the things that upset me. But it just makes me mad at him that I can't.

Anger is often self-directed. As caregivers increasingly realize their inability to prevent the suffering of their loved ones, some will try to blame themselves for the advent of this situation. One gay man expressed it in this way: "I can't help it. I feel like it's my fault he has AIDS. I mean, maybe I gave it to him! I know there's no way to tell but I still feel that way." Another, the ex-wife of an AIDS-diagnosed recovering addict, blames herself: "If I had just stayed with him and helped him fight the drugs. Then maybe he wouldn't be sick. I still love him, so I don't know why I left him."

As caregivers compare notes during group meetings, it becomes evident that quality of care, depth of knowledge, and doctor-patient rapport can all vary significantly. It is not surprising that a frequent target for anger within the group is the medical community. As Kastenbaum and Aisenberg (1972, p. 418), noted, "Most Americans . . . cannot remember a time when 'wonder drugs' (already an archaic term) did not figure prominently in their physician's armamentarium. . . . Not only were the treatments usually effective, but they were doled out lovingly by mother." The bitter truth that PWAs and their caregivers are facing is that there is no wonder drug. As often as not, the individual doctor must inform the patient that the potential treatment can be as devastating as the disease.

Some symptoms simply defy treatment. For others, the medical community must admit to a paucity of knowledge. Caregivers' awareness that the willingness of a doctor to monitor a patient on an experimental drug or novel therapy can be a life or death decision can often put caregivers and their loved ones in direct conflict with the medical establishment. The result often is doctor and hospital shopping.

One woman recounted the experience her son had in finding a doctor to treat him: "He had called three doctors recommended by his HMO. When he described his symptoms, all three claimed they weren't taking new patients. Finally he wised up and lied about symptoms just to get in to a doctor so he could be treated." Because the group is open-ended, and the course of the disease like a roller coaster, the resurgence of anger in group meetings is a frequent event. Indeed, the opportunity to vent angry feelings appears to be a primary benefit of group membership. One result of the uneven medical care people receive is that the group begins to act as an informal referral network for group members, and it is this particular support that helps members begin to take control of their situations. The anger at the medical establishment serves as a motivator to do something, and members often begin a frenzy of political activities, speaking engagements, or educational initiatives with other family members, professionals, and colleagues at work.

DEPRESSION

As the period of care lengthens, caregivers begin to experience frequent depression as they attempt to cope with AIDS-related problems on a daily basis. The caprice and inconsistencies posed by AIDS make short-term planning a questionable venture. Financial resources are often strained to the breaking point after repeated hospitalizations. The cost of life-sustaining drugs can run into thousands of dollars per year. It may be impossible to bring in help to care for the patient while the caregiver is at work, placing an added burden of worry on the caregiver. Traditional sources of care often are viewed with distrust. One woman, a schoolteacher in a small town, recounts: "I didn't dare use the local visiting nurses while I was at work. The town is just too small, and I just couldn't risk it getting out that my husband had AIDS." Her solution was to call home during her workday, as frequently as possible, to check on him.

STRIKING A BALANCE

The bouts of denial, anger, and depression that the caregivers experienced were not always predictable. Their occurrence and frequency followed the roller coaster progress of the disease itself. What has become apparent is that some caregivers vacillate between anger and depression and seem at times to give up on group support, as it really does not change the physical status of the PWA. Other members seem to adopt a realistic appraisal of the impending finality of the disease. Perhaps it is the repeated hospitalizations with bouts of life-endangering infections that prompt this attitude. One mother in the group expressed these feelings: "This time [when my son was hospitalized], I realized he might die there. Ever since then, every time something happens, I tell myself that this could be it. I'm resigned to his death. I don't know how he goes on fighting." Although accepting the possible death of their charges, most caregivers arrive at an attitude that allows them to take each day in its turn: "I try to be hopeful that some new therapy or drug will turn up. Mostly I just try to enjoy the time we have together," said a spouse. Other caregivers expressed a sense of regret for lost time or opportunities. Another spouse said, "When I think of the amount of time I've wasted, it kills me. But I can't have it back. I have to make sure that the time we have left is the best possible I can provide." Still others found a sense of renewed opportunities; one spouse noted, "I feel like I say things and feelings I wouldn't have before. I'm more honest with my lover now."

The group reinforces development of this attitude. Incoming members see it constantly manifested by the "old-timers." New members will often try strategies suggested and proven valid by the more experienced members. Regardless of the experience, the message from the group to the individual member stresses quality of life. The climate is one of encouragement, reassurance, and the striking of a balance between fighting the odds and facing reality. We feel the support of the group is essential in reducing caregivers' uncertainties, fears, and worries and helping them provide the most important part of the PWAs' care.

CONCLUSION

New issues arise and old ones take new forms as the disease moves toward chronicity. Despite identifying and dealing with anger continuously, at one meeting a veteran member complained, "There is no place for anger in *this* group." This may be explained in several ways. There appears to be a variety of angers extant within the group. The anger this father refers to is more diffuse and less identifiable. The more easily verbalized feeling of anger is associated with specific events: the person with AIDS has a setback or is the victim of a mistake, discrimination, or some real slight on the part of the society. In this context, the caregiver's anger is directed at an object, it can be specifically identified, its cause described, and a planned reaction to the circumstances can be designed and discussed.

A form of anger that is not easily worked through has been labeled "volatile emotions" (Peppers and Knapp 1980) in some of the literature. This is more of a rage that is undirected, consisting of physical violence and/or verbal outbursts. It is the extreme expression of helplessness. This rage is difficult for others to witness, as it increases their own anxiety. The message to those who feel this way is that it is not acceptable to vent these feelings.

Another consideration is that, as the number of caregivers seeking services has increased, an influx of new members has entered the group. These new members may be in the premature burying stage while veteran members are experiencing anger. The possibility exists that, as veterans reconstruct their lives, they are concerned about the fragile state of the new members and hesitant to discuss what they see in store for them.

A third possibility is that, although there has been increased education about AIDS, stigmatizing of the disease continues. As families recognize that AIDS is no longer a crisis that will end within a year or two, their anger turns to rage.

AIDS has become a chronic disease and, although traditional social service agencies showed some interest in providing care when there was the possibility of federal financial support, this was short-lived. Grass-root projects have had to continue providing care for both PWAs and their loved ones. The volunteer base has become fatigued and has not always been able to change views of client and family strains necessitated by the changing form of AIDS, now a chronic illness. What began as crisis intervention is not adequate for long-term care.

Despite the increased need of PWAs and their families for social support, it is unlikely that new services will be forthcoming. Public resources continue to be scarce (Chachkes 1987) and the responsibility for planning a coordinated response continues to be placed on families and grass root organizations. However, the focus of services needs to change. More in-depth support to both PWAs and their caregivers must be offered. PWAs must be viewed in a social network, making it essential that we include the nonprofessional caregivers in our thinking as we reorganize services and ponder the social implications of this disease. Agencies serving PWAs must view caregivers in a dual role. They are at once clients, who have psychosocial needs, and service providers, in need of concrete advice and information to manage ongoing care. Although organizations have recognized the caregiver's need for information and advice, they have failed to provide for the emotional needs of people giving care on an ongoing basis. Other organizations have recognized and responded to this dual need but have been unable to keep up with the expanded needs of families caused by a disease that has changed from a crisis to a chronic illness.

Research needs to be continually updated on the social dilemmas created for PWAs and their caregivers as the disease takes on new forms. As medical discoveries continue to be advanced, and political and social messages to the public are reconstructed, it is likely there will be new problems for both these groups. Concomitant with the increasing number of persons living with AIDS, the cost will rise for research and for sustaining care. The possibility of an exponential increase of individuals who are permanently disabled, supported by public funds and requiring expensive ongoing medical care will add to the competition for shrinking dollars with others who suffer from different life-threatening illnesses. Political frustration with the need for increased expenditures will raise new ethical problems concerning where monies should be spent.

Prior to the development of increasingly successful prophylactic drugs (AZT, ddI, Bactrim Pentamidine, Dapsone, and so on), an HIV diagnosis was a death sentence. Expanding therapies and medical interventions have increased hopes that AIDS is becoming a treatable chronic disease. The caregivers of PWAs often find themselves in a shadowland of fearful hope. The end result is a psychological double bind. Most caregivers of terminally ill persons will experience a period of anticipatory grief (Charmaz 1980); the caregiver of a PWA is likely to experience repeated bouts of this, as life-threatening illnesses are contracted and fought off by the loved one. The emotional costs of dealing with the ebb and flow of anticipating death and expecting to continue the struggle for life are enormous. If we are to survive this epidemic, we must be sensitive to these emotional inconsistencies while being flexible and dynamic in our provision of care and support.

REFERENCES

Anderson, Robert and Michael Bury, eds. 1988. *Living With Chronic Illness.* Winchester, MA: Allen and Unwin.

Appleby, George and Barbara Sosnowitz. 1988. "Social Service Inaction Leads to Voluntary Response to AIDS." Presented to the National Association of Social Workers, Connecticut Chapter.

Bury, Michael. 1988. "Meanings at Risk: The Experience of Arthritis." Pp. 89-116 in *Living With Chronic Illness* edited by R. Anderson and M. Bury. Winchester, MA: Allen and Unwin.

Chachkes, Esther. 1987. "Women and Children With AIDS." Pp. 51-64 in *Responding to AIDS,* edited by C. Leukefeld and M. Fimbres. Silver Spring, MD: National Association of Social Workers.

Charmaz, Kathy. 1980. *The Social Reality of Death.* Reading, MA: Addison-Wesley.

Cogswell, Betty. 1968. "Some Structural Properties Influencing Socialization." *Administrative Science Quarterly* 13:417-40.

———. 1976. "Conceptual Model of Family as a Group: Family Response to Disability." Pp. 139-68 in *The Sociology of Physical Disability and Rehabilitation,* edited by G. Albrecht. Pittsburgh: University of Pittsburgh Press.

Crawford, Robert. 1986. "Individual Responsibility and Health Politics." Pp. 369-77 in *The Sociology of Health and Illness,* edited by P. Conrad and R. Kern. 2nd ed. New York: St. Martin's.

Hurwitz, Nathan. 1976. "The Origins of the Peer Self-Help Psychotherapy Group Movement." *Journal of Applied Behavioral Science* 12:283-94.

Kasl, Stanislav. 1983 "Social and Psychological Factors Affecting the Course of Disease: An Epidemiological Perspective." Pp. 683-708 in *Handbook of Health, Health Care and the Health Professions,* edited by D. Mechanic. New York: Free Press.

Kastenbaum, Robert and Ruth Aisenberg. 1972. *Psychology of Death.* New York: Springer.

Kelly, Jeffrey, Janet St. Lawrence, Steve Smith, Jr., Harold V. Hood, and Donna Cook. 1987. "Stigmatization of AIDS Patients by Physicians." *American Journal of Public Health* 77:789-91.

Knowles, John. 1986. "The Responsibility of the Individual." Pp. 358-68 in *The Sociology of Health and Illness,* edited by P. Conrad and R. Kern. 2nd ed. New York: St. Martin's.

Levitt, Eugene and Albert Klassen. 1979. "Public Attitudes Toward Homosexuality." Pp. 19-35 in *Gay Men: The Sociology of Male-Homosexuality,* edited by M. Levine. New York: Harper & Row.

Patton, Cindy. 1985. *Sex and Germs: The Politics of AIDS.* Boston: South End Press.

Peppers, Larry and Ronald Knapp. 1980. *Motherhood and Mourning.* New York: Praeger.

Pinder, Ruth. 1988. "Striking Balances: Living With Parkinson's Disease." Pp. 67-88 in *Living With Chronic Illness* edited by R. Anderson and M. Bury. Winchester, MA: Allen and Unwin.

Robinson, Ian. 1988. "Reconstructing Lives: Negotiating the Meaning of Multiple Sclerosis." Pp. 43-66 in *Living with Chronic Illness* edited by R. Anderson and M. Bury. Winchester, MA: Allen and Unwin.

Schneider, Beth. 1984. "Peril and Promise: Lesbians' Workplace Participation." Pp. 215-26 in *Feminist Frontiers,* edited by L. Richardson and V. Taylor. New York: Random House.

Sosnowitz, Barbara and George Appleby. 1988. "Preventing Volunteer Burn Out Through a Structured Support Network." Presented to the Society for the Study of Social Problems. Atlanta. August.

Strauss, Anselm and Barney Glaser. 1975. *Chronic Illness and the Quality of Life.* St. Louis: C. V. Mosby.

Taylor, Shelly, Roberta Falke, Steven Shoptaw, and Rosemary Lichtman. 1986. "Social Support, Support Groups, and the Cancer Patient." *Journal of Consulting and Clinical Psychology* 54:608-15.

8

Forced Blood Testing:
Role Taking, Identity, and Discrimination

Michael L. Schwalbe
Clifford L. Staples

Successful implementation of humane policies for dealing with AIDS and persons with AIDS depends on Americans' willingness to respond in a humane way to problems created by the disease. It is thus important to understand how people respond to AIDS-related policy dilemmas to develop effective education programs to encourage fairness and comparison.

Sociologists and others have already done much to document people's knowledge of and attitudes toward the disease AIDS (Altman 1986; Brandt 1986; Casper 1986; Eisenberg 1986; Simkins and Kushner 1986; Katz et al. 1987; O'Donnell, O'Donnell, Pleck, Snarey, and Rose 1987; Temoshok, Sweet, and Zich 1987; DiClemente, Boyer, and Morales 1988). There also has been some research, mostly in the form of opinion polls, on people's attitudes toward various proposals for public policies to deal with AIDS (see *Gallup Report,* June 1987; Singer, Rogers, and Corcoran 1987). Research of this type is useful as social accounting; it tells us who knows what about the disease and who prefers to do what about it. But it is important to know more than the conclusions people have arrived at or the attitudes they have formed. We need to examine the social psychological dynamics that underlie people's responses to AIDS-related policy proposals (see Berk 1987; Nelkin 1987).

Our concern is with what underlies people's responses to the conflicts of interests and values that AIDS has generated. In our view, the most interesting judgments people must make about AIDS policies involve instances in which group interests conflict or moral principles clash. It is in attempting to resolve such conflicts that people must truly make judgments, not simply express opinions. What we are thus interested in here are people's judgments about the acceptability of courses of action that serve some interests while sacrificing others. These are dilemmas in the sense that there is no solution that serves all interests and values equally well.

At this time in U.S. history, the appearance of AIDS has given rise to a multitude of such dilemmas. Our cultural milieu encompasses militant homosexuality as well as intense homophobia; an obsession with sexuality, fueled by advertising, as well as an inability to publicly discuss explicitly sexual matters; a strong hope that scientists will soon discover a cure for the disease as well as a widespread distrust of experts; a secular, scientific view of disease as well as a religiously based punishment conception of disease. We also lack recent experience in dealing with deadly epidemics. In this context of divergent values and beliefs, and of limited technical knowledge, nearly all AIDS policies have entailed some kind of moral dilemma.

To understand the judgments people make when faced with an AIDS-related dilemma, we must do more than document these judgments or correlate them with demographic variables. We need a theoretical framework that can begin to account for the process in which judgments are formed. That is part of what we attempt to provide in this chapter, which reports the results of a research project intended to document the effects of factual knowledge, self-conceptions, and role-taking abilities on judgments about an AIDS-related policy dilemma. We draw on the social psychology of G. H. Mead ([1908] 1964, 1934) to account for the importance of these variables and the mechanisms by which they affect people's judgments.

THEORETICAL BACKGROUND

We begin from the premise that most action is habitual; that is, it does not involve conscious reflection on means in relation to ends. Such action proceeds smoothly until a problem is encountered, at which point reflection is required. AIDS-related policy dilemmas are such problems for two reasons. First, this is because AIDS-related dilemmas by definition entail conflicting values and interests that "pull action in two directions at once," hence bringing action to a halt until some reconciliation is achieved. Second, this is because the policy problems that AIDS has created are largely unfamiliar ones for which we have no ready-made solutions. Thus we are again forced to stop and try to discover a new way past the problem.

As a society, we have thus been forced by a virus to confront the inadequacies of our traditional modes of action. The problems the disease has created have forced us to reflect and debate about how to reconcile a whole new set of conflicts between the values and interests of individuals and groups. Not all of the reflection and debate that feed into the problem-solving process occur in highly visible public arenas. Much of it occurs privately, in everyday life, as individuals reflect upon the problems AIDS has forced upon them and upon others they know. Our interest is in the characteristics of the individual that influence this reflection.

Various theories of moral cognition attempt to specify what it is that individuals must take into account when trying to solve moral problems. Several parallel theoretical traditions (see Vine 1983; Kohlberg 1984; Rest 1986) propose models of moral reasoning that suggest reasoning typically includes consideration of the facts of the situation; one's own interests, values, and self-esteem needs; and the perspectives of others. Meadian social psychology, upon which we draw, also emphasizes the importance of these aspects of moral cognition.

Mead's social psychology also is the basis for his ethical theory, which is concerned with how moral problems—conflicts over which ends to pursue—should be resolved (see Mead [1908] 1964, 1934, pp. 379-89). So it will be appropriate here to discuss both aspects of Mead's thinking together. In Mead's view, the first step toward finding a solution to a moral problem is to impartially consider the facts that define its existence; these facts include the values, interests, thoughts, and feelings of all stakeholders in the situation. Ignoring any such facts would be morally irresponsible. Though facts alone will not necessarily lead to discovery of the best possible solution, their consideration is essential to the process.

Pertinent knowledge of the situation includes knowledge of others. Much of this knowledge must be obtained through role taking. It is only by taking the role of the others whose values and interests are at stake in the problematic situation that the individual can discover the facts relevant to finding a workable solution. Those who would attempt to solve moral problems, to resolve dilemmas, must, therefore, be inclined to take the perspectives of others (see Kohlberg 1973). Competent moral problem solvers, in Mead's view, must have both a propensity to role take and the developed ability to do so.

Not only must moral problem solvers take the perspectives of others, they must also reflect on their own values and interests, for these are no less relevant to the situation. Moreover, some values and beliefs are of particular importance in determining how people will decide to act in problematic situations. Beliefs about the self and the values attached to those beliefs are especially consequential. In general, people will strive to act in ways that protect and preserve their most cherished beliefs about themselves (see Rokeach 1973, 1985). What are, therefore, also important to consider in a problematic situation are people's identities and self-conceptions (see Gilligan 1987).

What we are developing here is a model that specifies the characteristics of the individual that should be consequential for producing judgments about policy dilemmas. These characteristics are knowledge, self-conceptions, and role-taking abilities. This, of course, presumes dilemmas of a particular kind: those in which values and interests of different persons are recognized to conflict. In such cases, judgments should depend on (a) factual knowledge of the situation, (b) the individual's self-conceptions, and (c) the individual's inclination and ability to take the role of others in the situation. The disease AIDS, with its mysterious biological character, its perceived association with deviant sexuality, and its sheer deadliness, seems especially likely to demand judgments that implicate these aspects of social psychological functioning (see Last 1987; Mohr 1987a, 1987b; Valdiserri 1987).

The problem that remains, of course, is determining precisely what sort of knowledge, which self-conceptions, and what kinds of role-taking abilities are most important. These are properly matters for discovery. But to afford a preliminary test of our model, we have assessed the types of knowledge, self-conceptions, and role-taking abilities that seem, on the surface, to be most relevant to making judgments about AIDS-related policy dilemmas.

We will thus be looking at the effects of (a) factual knowledge about the disease, (b) the strength of the moral self-concept, (c) role-taking propensity, (d) role-taking accuracy, (e) role-taking range, and (f) role-taking depth on people's tendencies to agree or disagree with actions taken in response to AIDS-related problems. Moreover, by taking these variables into account simultaneously, we will be able to make some determinations of their relative importance. We believe that this sort of analysis is essential to identifying what are likely to be the most effective strategies for promoting just, compassionate, and life-saving public policies with regard to AIDS. Formulating such policies will depend on knowing what is most powerfully affecting people's thinking about the disease and about the moral dilemmas it creates.

METHODS

Sample

Data from this study derive from questionnaires administered to undergraduates in introductory sociology courses during spring 1988 at a medium-sized university in the upper Midwest. Students were offered extra credit for participation, though this did not significantly affect participation rates; after explanation of the project's purpose and assurance of anonymity, few students chose not to fill out the questionnaire. The resulting sample of 443 respondents was 52% female and 48% male, with a mean age of 20.0 years. Participants also were predominantly single/never married (93%), white (95%), and self-described as heterosexual (93%) or celibate (6%). About half grew up in small towns. More than a third reported attending church at least once a week, 36% reported attending once a month, and 26% reported once or twice a year or not at all.

Measures

Our independent variables are knowledge about the disease AIDS, role-taking propensity, role-taking accuracy, role-taking range, role-taking depth, and moral self-conceptions. Measurement procedures for each variable are described in turn below (see the Appendix for further details).

Knowledge about the disease AIDS was measured using a nine-item true/false test. The following are examples of items: "AIDS is caused by a virus"; AIDS can be transmitted from a mother to her unborn child"; and "AIDS can be contracted through giving blood." The number of correct answers was summed into a knowledge-of-AIDS index score.

Role-taking propensity is an individual's characteristic readiness to take the perspectives of others. Our measure of role-taking propensity is adapted from the empathic responsiveness subscale of Bernstein and

Davis's (1982) Interpersonal Reactivity Index. It includes four self-descriptive statements implicitly referring to role-taking tendencies (e.g., "Sometimes I'm just not interested in trying to see things from the other person's point of view"), for which respondents were asked to indicate on a 4-point, Likert-type scale how well it described them (*not very well at all* to *very well*). Item responses were summed into a role-taking propensity scale score.

We use the concepts of role-taking range, accuracy, and depth as developed by Schwalbe (1988). Briefly, *role-taking range* refers to the extent of an individual's ability to adopt multiple perspectives. *Accuracy* refers to an individual's ability to correctly discern the response tendencies of others in particular situations. *Depth* refers to the extent to which an individual can grasp the perceptions and motivations of another. In this formulation, role-taking ability is seen as varying in multiple dimensions, and each dimension of ability is distinguished from the propensity to apply it. The measures described below are first attempts to measure the constructs.

Range was measured by asking subjects to indicate the strength of their agreement (on a 4-point, Likert-type scale) with statements such as "I could never understand why someone would become a communist," and "I think I could understand why someone would want to join a religious group and live in a monastery." Responses to five items were summed to create a score for role-taking range. Accuracy was measured using the same strategy. Respondents were asked to indicate on a 4-point scale their agreement with statements such as "I am often surprised by how people respond to me in face-to-face encounters," and "I can usually predict how my friends will react to things in any given situation." Responses to five such items were summed to create a score for role-taking accuracy.[1]

To measure depth, subjects were presented with two brief vignettes in which a student was described as behaving in some unusual and unexplained way (see the Appendix). They were then asked to give as many plausible reasons as they could think of to account for the behavior described in the vignette. Our measure of role-taking depth is the number of the discrete reasons subjects offered to account for the behaviors described in both vignettes.

We conceptualize the moral self-concept as an individual's evaluation of him- or herself as a morally responsible actor. We do not see this as a specific identity (i.e., "I am a moral person") but as a general evaluation that derives from self-perceptions of tendencies to act in ways that are culturally defined as good or bad. To measure this construct, we asked subjects to indicate how well (on a 4-point, Likert-type scale) they were described by a series of statements that referred to various kinds of moral action (e.g., "I always avoid causing harm to others"; "I follow agreed-upon rules and meet my obligations to the group"). We created a moral self-concept score for each respondent by summing the responses for each of these four items.

Two other independent variables, religiosity and sex, which were also included for control purposes, were measured using standard demographic items.

Our dependent variable is a judgment about the correctness of an action taken in response to an AIDS-related moral dilemma. The dilemma we created involved discrimination against workers by the management of a food processing plant. We presented half of our subjects with one version of the vignette, and the remaining subjects were presented with a different version. The first vignette read as follows:

> The chief manager of a food processing plant ordered several male employees who were known to be gay to submit to testing for exposure to the AIDS virus. The manager said this was necessary to protect the company's public image, upon which its profitability depended. The employees, who were all performing well in their jobs, refused to take the tests, arguing that they were being discriminated against illegally. They also argued that employees who were not openly gay were not being targeted for testing. Lawyers for the company advised the manager that firing the openly gay employees for not submitting to the tests would indeed be illegal. The manager decided not to risk a lawsuit and got rid of the employees anyway by reorganizing the departments in which they worked so that their jobs were eliminated.

We call this version "Gay Objectors." The second version describes the same type of situation, except there is no mention of sexual preference, and the third sentence has been changed to read: "Several employees, who were all performing well in their jobs, refused to take the tests, arguing that they were being discriminated against illegally since managers and front office workers were exempt from the testing." The manager's response is the same: the dissident workers, whose sexuality is not specified, are gotten rid of through departmental reorganization. We call this version "Objectors."

We thus have two cases of AIDS-related discrimination, but, in the first case, those who are discriminated against are known to be gay, whereas, in the second case, the workers' sexuality is unspecified. This procedure, inspired by the factorial design approach to measuring social judgments developed by Rossi and Nock (1982), allows us to address the important question of whether our subjects are more willing to approve of AIDS-related discrimination against gays than against others. Each question-naire contained only one version of the vignette, either "Gay Objectors" or "Objectors." They were randomly assigned to subjects simply by alternating the questionnaires as they were distributed. Subjects were not aware that there were two different versions of the vignette.

In each case, subjects were asked to indicate on a 5-point, Likert-type scale how strongly they agreed with the action taken by the manager. We take agreement to be an indication of concurrence of judgment, effec-tively equivalent to indicating that the action described was the right action to take. Responses to the agree/disagree question constitute our dependent variable.

RESULTS

We first turn to the question of whether or not our subjects were more willing to approve of discrimination against gays than against others. Unfortunately, the answer is yes. As Table 8.1 indicates, those who read "Gay Objectors" were significantly more likely to agree with the man-ager's actions than were those who read "Objectors." Although, overall, subjects were not inclined to agree with the discriminatory actions of the manager—both means were below 2.0 on the 5-point scale—when vic-tims of the discrimination were identifiably gay, support for the manager's actions was substantially stronger. Thus, among these college students, discrimination against gays in an AIDS-related dilemma was apparently more acceptable than discrimination against others.

Because there is some evidence that men, particularly young, hetero-sexual, college men (see Kurdek 1988; Herek 1984), are inclined to express extremely negative (i.e., "homophobic") attitudes toward gays, we wanted to determine whether the greater support for the manager in the "Gay Objectors" vignette was specifically attributable to the male subjects. The cell means shown in Table 8.2 appear to confirm this suspicion. Although the 124 women who read "Gay Objectors" were only slightly more likely to approve of the manager's actions than were the 105 women who read "Objectors," the 101 men who read "Gay Objectors" were much more likely than the 113 men who read *Objectors* to approved of the manager's actions. This apparent effect of the interaction between

Table 8.1 t-Test on Mean Differences for Gay Objectors
Versus Objectors

	Number of Cases	Mean[a]	Standard Deviation	Standard Error
Gay objectors	225	1.45	1.37	.091
Objectors	218	.94	1.13	.076

a. Scale range = 0 (strongly disagree) to 4 (strongly agree).
b. t value = 4.30; df = 441; two-tailed probability = .000.

being male and the mention of gay sexuality holds up throughout our analysis.

Table 8.3 presents the correlation matrix upon which the remainder of the analysis is based. Listwise deletion of missing data reduced the sample size to 406. Because there are a number of significant correlations among the independent variables, we used multiple regression analysis to explore the relationship between these variables and our dependent variable, agreement with the manager's actions. Table 8.4 presents the results of this analysis. The equation includes all of the independent variables discussed above, plus a sex × vignette interaction term, as the cell means in Table 8.2 suggested would be appropriate. The equation accounts for a significant proportion of the variation in judgments about the manager's actions (R^2 = .169, p < .001), and 4 of the 10 independent variables have effects that are significant beyond the .05 level. As our preliminary analysis would lead us to expect, the sex × vignette interaction is significant and relatively strong (Beta = .285). Again, the effect of being male and knowing that the dissident workers were gay resulted in an almost one-point shift (B = .884) toward agreement with the manager, other things being equal.

Table 8.2 Mean Differences by Sex and Vignette for Agreement with Manager

Objectors		Gay Objectors	
Men (113)	Women (105)	Men (101)	Women (124)
.93	.94	1.92	1.06

NOTE: Scale range = 0 (strongly disagree) to 4 (strongly agree).

Table 8.3 Correlation Matrix for All Variables

	RTP	RTA	RTR	RTD	MSC	KNO	SEX	VIG	REL
RTP	—								
RTA	.124*	—							
RTR	.379**	.140*	—						
RTD	.013	.049	.062	—					
MSC	.262**	.180**	.183**	.007	—				
KNO	.055	.055	.077	-.055	.059	—			
SEX	-.228**	.004	-.079	-.132*	-.264**	.042	—		
VIG	-.038	-.012	-.074	.053	.043	-.054	-.079	—	
REL	.142*	-.013	.118*	.026	.111	-.093	-.038	.042	—
AGR	-.148*	-.045	-.205**	.004	-.188**	-.105	.167**	.196**	.111

NOTE: RTP = role-taking propensity; RTA = role-taking accuracy; RTR = role-taking range; RTD = role-taking depth; MSC = moral self-concept; KNO = knowledge about AIDS; SEX = "being male"; VIG = gay objectors; REL = religiosity; AGR = agreement with manager's action.

Of the four role-taking variables, only role-taking range was significant (Beta = -.152). Greater range was associated, as we might expect, with reduced support for the discriminatory behavior of the manager. Moral self-concept was also a significant predictor (Beta = -.112), a strong

Table 8.4 Equation Predicting Agreement with Actions of Manager

Independent Variables	Dependent Variable: "Agree with Manager"	
	B	Beta
R-T propensity	-.020	-.052
R-T accuracy	.000	.012
R-T range	-.082	-.152*
R-T depth	.000	.000
AIDS knowledge	-.092	-.082
Moral self-concept	-.082	-.113*
Religiosity	.172	.134*
Sex[a]	-.092	-.036
Vignette[b]	.040	.016
Sex × vignette	.885	.285**
R^2 .169**		

a. Female = 0; male = 1.
b. Objectors = 0; gay objectors = 1.
*$p < .05$; **$p < .001$.

moral self-concept being associated with reduced support for the manager's actions. In contrast, religiosity had a positive effect (Beta = .133): the more frequent the church attendance, the greater the support for the manager. Finally, it is worth noting that, although AIDS knowledge does not quite reach the conventional level of significance (p = .079), the effect was in the expected direction—greater knowledge about the disease reduced support for the manager (Beta = -.082).

DISCUSSION AND CONCLUSIONS

We have looked at some of the social psychological dynamics underlying people's judgments about a dilemma associated with the disease AIDS—a dilemma that pitted the civil rights of workers against a company's right to protect its profitability. We found, overall, that college students were willing to give only mild support to a manager who discriminated against workers by firing them for refusing to submit to a blood test. However, we also found that men, but not women, were much more willing to support the discriminatory behavior of the manager when the workers in question were known to be gay.

Our attempt to predict support for the manager with a model derived from Mead's social psychology was only partially successful; only two of the six theoretically relevant variables were statistically significant. We observed, not surprisingly, that role-taking range and a conception of oneself as a moral actor diminished the tendency to agree with discriminatory action of the manager. This suggests that the ability to role take with a wide range of others, as well as the tendency to define oneself in moral terms, are important to understanding resistance to discrimination and are also likely to be important in predicting preference for humane AIDS policies. On the other hand, none of the role-taking propensity, role-taking accuracy, or role-taking depth variables had a significant effect on the subjects' willingness to support or not support the manager. Knowledge about the disease did diminish the tendency to discriminate, though the effect was small and not statistically significant at the .05 level.

At this point, it is worth considering further the most important, and most disturbing, finding: the sex × vignette interaction. The willingness of these young college men, but not their female classmates, to approve of the manager's discriminatory actions only when the victims of the repression were known to be gay is consistent with the growing number of accounts of intolerance and outright violence toward gays that have occurred in the wake of the AIDS epidemic in the United States (Walter 1986). Although the public has never approved of equal rights for gays (see de Boer 1978), the desire of the largely white, heterosexual majority to shield itself both physically and socially from the disease has provided a climate of social approval for "gay bashing." If our findings here can be generalized, male homophobia is the root cause of this trend and, as such, may also be the primary impediment to the implementation of humane public policies toward AIDS.

Although accounting for male homophobia is beyond the scope of this chapter, it seems appropriate to suggest how it might be linked to our theoretical analysis. Our view is that male homophobia stems in large part from the threat male homosexuality poses to traditional masculine identity. The argument, briefly, is that masculine identity is experienced not only in terms of difference from feminine identity but in terms of *superiority* to it (Pleck 1981); that masculine superiority is maintained in part through sexual practice (Dworkin 1981); that male homosexuality blurs the male/female boundary normally maintained through heterosexual and sexual practice (MacKinnon 1987); hence, male homosexuality is consciously or unconsciously perceived as a threat to male dominance (Brittan 1989). This argument is also supported by considerable evidence that male homophobia is closely linked to support for traditional gender roles (see Lehne 1989 for a review).

It may thus be that many men fear or are angered by the prospect of equal rights for gays because this threatens a core identity—heterosexual male—and the system of gender relations that sustains this identity. But because heterosexual women do not benefit as men do from this system, it is understandable that they are less prone to feel threatened by male homosexuality. The case of heterosexual male homophobia is thus less mysterious if one sees that the threat heterosexual men experience is not to their dominance over gay men but to dominance over heterosexual women. Support for the discriminatory actions of the manager in the "Gay Objectors" vignette was perhaps a response to this threat.

If we view our variable "sex" as a proxy for gender identity, our findings and interpretation are consistent with Meadian social psychology. As discussed earlier, the Meadian view sees a person's self-conceptions as crucial to moral decision making. Typically, gender identity is a core self-conception. And, as we also discussed earlier, people will tend to act in ways that preserve these most central beliefs about the self. By supporting the manager's actions, the men in our sample were perhaps attempting to protect an important identity they felt would be threatened by allowing gay men equal rights. Women apparently did not feel particularly threatened by the fact that the workers were known to be gay and, therefore, did not support discrimination against the gay men. In both cases, it seems that identities played an important part in shaping responses to this moral dilemma.

What we have tried to show here is something of the social psychological complexity underlying people's judgments about AIDS-related policy dilemmas. These judgments are clearly not the simple product of straightforward reasoning based on incontrovertible facts. To a great extent, people's self-conceptions and their role-taking abilities will determine how the facts are perceived and processed. It is not that factual knowledge is irrelevant, but it seems to be less relevant in determining what people will tolerate (by way of repressive policies) than who people are and what they want to believe about themselves and others, particularly deviant others. The key, then, to understanding how people arrive at judgments about AIDS-related policy dilemmas may lie in determining which interests and self-conceptions they feel are threatened by particular policy options.

The above discussion suggests a few directions for future research on this problem. First, to test our post hoc theorizing here, it would be necessary to collect additional data that include, in place of sex, a measure of gender identity. Although a variable that measures a person's support for traditional gender roles would suffice, one that measures more precisely the extent to which a heterosexual's gender role, and sexuality, revolve around power would be ideal. Such a measure would allow a more precise assessment of the impact that gender identity has on AIDS-related policy dilemmas in general and on AIDS-related policy dilemmas that involve gays in particular.

Finally, we hope this study will encourage further investigation of what affects judgments about AIDS-related dilemmas. It would be interesting to reproduce this analysis with other populations, particularly politicians, health care providers (see Richardson, Lochner, McGuigan, and Levine 1987; Katz et al. 1987; Kim and Perfect 1988), and the general public. A wider range of dilemmas could also be presented to determine what activates particular values and self-conceptions among different groups of people. Our analysis also suggests that it would be interesting to challenge people's self-conceptions in experimental situations and then test for changes in patterns of judgment about AIDS-related dilemmas. Specifically, a "self-confrontation" (see Rokeach 1973, 1985; Greenstein 1989) procedure might be used to reduce levels of male homophobia and thereby diminish the tendency to discriminate against gays. In sum, future research should seek to determine not only what affects judgments in people as they are but how judgments might be changed to encourage support for scientifically sound and morally responsible policies.

APPENDIX:
ITEMS AND SCALES

Knowledge of AIDS Test Items

Answer the following questions either *true* or *false:*

1. Today, blood donations are no longer screened for evidence of AIDS infection. (F)
2. AIDS is caused by a virus. (T)
3. The use of condoms during sex greatly increases the risk of transmitting AIDS, though at present it is not known why this is so. (F)
4. There is no cure for AIDS. (T)
5. AIDS can be contracted through giving blood. (F)
6. As of December 1989, about 500,000 people had died of AIDS in the United States. (F)
7. In eastern Africa, AIDS has struck primarily homosexuals. (F)
8. AIDS can be transmitted from a mother to her unborn child. (T)
9. Research indicates that AIDS is not spread through casual contact, such as the sharing of a drinking glass. (T)

Score = number of correct; hypothetical range = 0-9; actual range = 2-9; mean correct = 7.2; *s.d.* = 1.15.

Role-Taking Propensity

Items describing subject *not very well at all* (= 0) to *very well* (= 3):

1. Sometimes I'm just not interested in trying to see things from the other person's point of view.
2. I try to look at everybody's side of the argument before I make up my mind.
3. Before judging what someone else says or does, I try to imagine how I would feel if I were in their shoes.

4. I try to understand other people's behavior by imagining how they see the world.

Hypothetical range = 0-12; actual range = 1-12; mean = 7.31; s.d. = 2.12; average interitem correlation = .253; alpha = .577.

Role-Taking Accuracy

Items describing subject *not very well at all* (= 0) to *very well* (= 3):

1. I am usually good at figuring out beforehand how others will react to what I'll say or do in a particular situation.
2. I can usually predict how my friends will react to things in any given situation.
3. Even in unusual situations, I'm usually able to figure out what's expected of me.

Hypothetical range = 0-9; actual range = 2-9; mean = 5.95; *s.d.* = 1.12; average interitem correlation = .279; alpha = .537.

Role-Taking Range

Items describing subject *not very well at all* (= 0) to *very well* (= 3):

1. I think I could understand why someone would want to join a religious group and live in a monastery.
2. I think the religious fanatics, like those in the Mideast, are just plain crazy.
3. I could never understand why someone would become a communist.
4. I can really appreciate the values and ideas of the hippies of the 1960s.

Hypothetical range = 0-12; actual range = 0-12; mean = 6.38; *s.d.* = 2.01; average iteritem correlation = .250; alpha = .504.

Role-Taking Depth

Total number of reasons given for actions described in both of the following scenarios:

1. A popular female student majoring in creative writing was doing well in all her courses and had only a year to go before graduation. In midyear she dropped out of school and moved to southern California, where she had no relatives. When she contacted her friends, she talked as if everything were normal but refused to explain why she quit school and moved.

2. The friends of a student majoring in business knew him to be bright and creative. But he would drink heavily the night before big exams and so was doing poorly in his courses. During his junior year his father died. After that he changed his major to philosophy, quit drinking before exams, and never received a grade lower than A- in any course.

More reasons = greater role-taking depth; range = 2-17; mean = 7.33; *s.d.* = 2.76.

Moral Self-Concept

Items describing subject *not very well at all* (= 0) to *very well* (= 3):

1. I always avoid causing harm to others.

2. I am pleasant and helpful to others.

3. I obey the law and am respectful of authority.

4. I follow agreed-upon rules and meet my obligations to the group.

Hypothetical range = 0-12; actual range = 3-12; mean = 9.19; *s.d.* = 1.29; alpha = .558.

NOTE

1. Role-taking accuracy is conceived as a situationally demonstrated ability. It depends on skill in perceiving and decoding signs of an other's subjective and objective worldviews (see Schwalbe 1988). A proper measure would then somehow seek to document the use of such skill in a variety of situations. The paper-and-pencil measures we use here are thus at best proxy indicators of role-taking abilities.

REFERENCES

Altman, Dennis. 1986. *AIDS in the Mind of America: The Social, Political, and Psychological Impact of a New Epidemic.* Garden City, NY: Anchor/Doubleday.

Berk, Richard A. 1987. "Anticipating the Social Consequences of AIDS: A Position Paper." *American Sociologist* 18:211-27.

Bernstein, William M. and Mark H. Davis. 1982. "Perspective-Taking, Self-Consciousness, and Accuracy in Person Perception." *Basic and Applied Social Psychology* 3:1-19.

Brandt, Allan. 1986. "AIDS: From Social History to Social Policy." *Law, Medicine, and Health Care* 14:231-42.

Brittan, Arthur. 1989. *Masculinity and Power.* Oxford: Basil Blackwell.

Casper, Virginia. 1986. "AIDS: A Psychosocial Perspective." Pp. 197-210 in *The Social Dimensions of AIDS: Method and Theory,* edited by D. A. Feldman and T. M. Johnson. New York: Praeger.

de Boer, Connie. 1978. "The Polls: Attitudes Toward Homosexuality." *Public Opinion Quarterly* 42:265-76.

DiClemente, Ralph J., Cherrie B. Boyer, and Edward S. Morales. 1988. "Minorities and AIDS: Knowledge, Attitudes, and Misconceptions Among Black and Latino Adolescents." *American Journal of Public Health* 78:55-57.

Dworkin, Andrea. 1981. *Pornography: Men Possessing Women.* London: Women's Press.

Eisenberg, Leon. 1986. "The Genesis of Fear: AIDS and the Public's Response to Science." *Law, Medicine, and Health Care* 14:243-49.

Gallup Report. June 1987. Report No. 261.

Gilligan, Carol. 1987. "Moral Orientation and Moral Development." Pp. 19-33 in *Women and Moral Theory,* edited by E. F. Kittay and D. T. Meyers. Totowa, NJ: Rowman & Littlefield.

Greenstein, Theodore. 1989. "Modifying Beliefs and Behavior Through Self-Confrontation." *Sociological Inquiry* 59:396-408.

Herek, Gregory M. 1984. "Beyond 'Homophobia': A Social Psychological Perspective on Attitudes Toward Lesbians and Gay Men." *Journal of Homosexuality* 10:1-21.

Katz, Irwin, R. Glen Hass, Nina Parisi, Janetta Astone, Denise McEvaddy, and David J. Lucido. 1987. "Lay People's and Health Care Personnel's Perception of Cancer, AIDS, Cardiac, and Diabetic Patients." *Psychological Reports* 60:615-29.

Kim, Jerome H. and John R. Perfect. 1988. "To Help the Sick: An Historical and Ethical Essay Concerning the Refusal to Care for Patients With AIDS." *American Journal of Medicine* 84:135-38.

Kohlberg, Lawrence. 1973. "The Claim to Moral Adequacy of a Highest Stage of Moral Judgment." *Journal of Philosophy* 70:630-46.

———. 1984. *Essays on Moral Development.* Vol. 2, *The Psychology of Moral Development.* New York: Harper & Row.

Kurdek, Lawrence A. 1988. "Correlates of Negative Attitudes Toward Homosexuals in Heterosexual College Students." *Sex Roles* 18:727-38.

Last, John M. 1987. Ethics, Mores and Values—and AIDS. *Canadian Journal of Public Health* 78:75-76.

Lehne, Gregory K. 1989. "Homophobia Among Men." Pp. 416-29 in *Men's Lives,* edited by M. S. Kimmel and M. A. Messner. New York: Macmillan.

MacKinnon, Catherine A. 1987. *Feminism Unmodified: Discourses on Life and Law.* Cambridge, MA: Harvard University Press.

Mead, George H. [1908] 1964. "The Philosophical Basis of Ethics." Pp. 82-93 in *Selected Writings, George Herbert Mead,* edited by A. J. Reck. New York: Bobbs-Merrill.

———. 1934. *Mind, Self and Society,* edited by C. W. Morris. Chicago: University of Chicago Press.

Mohr, Richard D. 1987a. "AIDS, Gays, and State Coercion." *Bioethics* 1:35-50.

———. 1987b. "Policy, Ritual, Purity: Gays and Mandatory AIDS Testing." *Law, Medicine, and Health Care* 15:178-85.

Nelkin, Dorothy. 1987. "AIDS and the Social Sciences: Review of Useful Knowledge and Research Needs." *Review of Infectious Disease* 9:980-86.

O'Donnell, Lydia, Carl O'Donnell, Joseph Pleck, John Snarey, and Richard M. Rose. 1987. "Psychosocial Responses of Hospital Workers to Acquired Immune Deficiency Syndrome." *Journal of Applied Social Psychology* 17:269-85.

Pleck, Joseph. 1981. *The Myth of Masculinity.* Cambridge: MIT Press.

Rest, James. 1986. *Moral Development: Advances in Research and Theory.* New York: Praeger.

Richardson, Jean L., Thomas Lochner, Kimberly McGuigan, and Alexandra M. Levine. 1987. "Physician Attitudes and Experience Regarding the Care of Patients With Acquired Immunodeficiency Syndrome and Related Disorders." *Medical Care* 25:675-85.

Rokeach, Milton. 1973. *The Nature of Human Values.* New York: Free Press.

———. 1982. *Value Survey*(Form G). Sunnyvale, CA: Halgren Tests.

———. 1985. "Inducing Change and Stability in Belief Systems and Personality Structure." *Journal of Social Issues* 41:153-71.

Rossi, Peter and Steven L. Nock. 1982. *Measuring Social Judgments: The Factorial Survey Approach.* Beverly Hills, CA: Sage.

Schwalbe, Michael L. 1988. "Role Taking Reconsidered: Linking Competence and Performance to Social Structure." *Journal for the Theory of Social Behavior.* 18:411-36.

Simkins, Lawrence and Aleen Kushner. 1986. "Attitudes Toward AIDS, Herpes II, and Toxic Shock Syndrome: Two Years Later." *Psychological Reports* 59:883-91.

Singer, Eleanor, Theresa Rogers, and Mary Corcoran. 1987. "AIDS." *Public Opinion Quarterly* 51:580-95.

Temoshek, Lydia, David M. Sweet, and Jane Zich. 1987. "The Three City Comparison of the Public's Knowledge of and Attitudes About AIDS." *Psychology and Health* 1:43-60.

Valdiserri, Ronald O. 1987. "Epidemics in Perspective." *Journal of Medical Humanities and Bioethics* 8:95-100.

Vine, Ian. 1983. "The Nature of Moral Commitments." Pp. 17-46 in *Morality in the Making: Thought, Action, and the Social Context,* edited by H. Weinreich-Haste and D. Jocke. New York: John Wiley.

9

Health Care
and the Social Construction of AIDS:
The Impact of Disease Definitions

Stephen Crystal
Marguerite Jackson

An important theme in the history of medicine and in medical sociology has been that diseases are socially constructed entities, not simply biological phenomena (Rosenberg 1988; Schneider and Conrad 1983; Cowie 1976; Mechanic 1978; Brandt 1985). This perception is eminently true of AIDS; such constructs shape societal and personal responses to the illness and, therefore, the experience of people with AIDS (McKinlay, Skinner, Riley, and Zablotsky 1989; Gilman 1988). One aspect of the social construction of AIDS that affects patients' experience involves disease

AUTHORS' NOTE: The Patient Subcommittee of the San Diego County Regional Task Force on AIDS (Rick Anderson, chair; Mark Herstand, co-chair) provided valuable information for development of the survey questions and was very helpful in distributing the questionnaires. We thank Eric Meyers and Nancy Fierro for interviewing PWAs and PWARCs; Angie Bartok (1986-87), Karen Zaustinsky (1989-90), Kathy Sowden (1989-90), and Michele Kleckner (1989-90) for data management; and the personnel of UCSD Medical Center Owen Clinic, the VA Medical Center, the San Diego AIDS Project, the AIDS Assistance Fund, the Center for Social Services/AIDS Response Program, the Urban League, the Fight Back Program, the San Diego County Department of Health Services Alternative Test Sites, and the other care providers for distribution of one or both surveys. We also are grateful to the University of California, San Diego, Academic Senate for financial assistance in the analysis of the 1986-87 survey and to the San Diego Community Healthcare Alliance and the United Way for funding the 1989-90 survey.

definitions that are, to some extent, medically arbitrary. The effect of such definitions is particularly important in a political culture in which the provision and financing of health care is particularistic rather than universal, where access to benefits and care systems depends on such specific characteristics of the individual as employment, family, disability, or income status.

Biologically, human immunodeficiency virus (HIV) infection brings about immunosuppression, which causes a spectrum of disease states (Institute of Medicine 1988). Socially, the experiences of illness is shaped by officially sanctioned but medically arbitrary categorizations of clinical syndromes within this spectrum (Oppenheimer 1988). Thus "official" AIDS, as defined by the Centers for Disease Control (CDC), requires the presence of certain marker conditions (Centers for Disease Control 1987). Persons "meeting criteria" for AIDS also are officially defined as "disabled," thus qualifying for various governmental health care and income benefits (Crystal and Jackson 1988). Others, whose HIV-associated illness may cause impairment of equal or greater severity, have been categorized as "pre-AIDS" or "AIDS-related complex" (ARC); (Institute of Medicine 1986) and more recently are referred to, even more ambiguously, as persons with "associated opportunistic infections" or "HIV-related illness" (Institute of Medicine 1988).

From the beginning of the epidemic, in terms of health care and social services needs, the focus was on CDC-defined AIDS. Indeed, this terminology is deeply embedded in the semantic referents we habitually employ. Our language incorporates a metaphorical figure of speech (formally known as synecdoche) in which the part is taken for the whole: The term *AIDS* has been habitually used when *HIV disease* is really meant. We tend to speak of the AIDS epidemic, AIDS health services, and so on; indeed, the title of this volume refers to the context of "AIDS." When we speak of *England* when referring to Great Britain, or *Russia* when referring to the Soviet Union, we may be led to think of these societies as less diverse than they really are. The consequences of the AIDS synecdoche are more significant. This sociolinguistic construction focuses our attention on the acute disease model of HIV illness; it leads the society to think in terms of a devastating, visible, acute, highly stigmatizing condition inevitably progressing to death over a relatively short period (Sontag 1989). Thus the language we use has kept the focus on persons dying of AIDS rather than on persons living with HIV. Our statistics, too, are shaped by medically arbitrary disease definition; we think in terms of the cases of CDC-defined AIDS reported in the United States to date, and included in surveillance statistics, rather than the larger number of individuals infected by the virus.

It is, however, in the area of health care and social benefit systems that the consequences of disease definitions are perhaps most concrete and most important. The current CDC AIDS case criterion (Centers for Disease Control 1987) is based on the surveillance definition developed for epidemiological monitoring purposes early in the epidemic, even before the cause of the syndrome was known. In case classification for epidemiological research on new and mystifying syndromes, it is more important to be specific than sensitive. Thus the definition is drawn narrowly rather than inclusively; it is more important to assure that all the cases being studied represent the same thing than to be sure that all the possible cases are included. The original CDC definition was expanded in 1987, but it is still the case that many individuals die of HIV without ever having been diagnosed with full-blown AIDS, and the definition leaves out many individuals with health care needs, as the data we discuss below demonstrate. Failure to include many individuals with severe illness, which persists even after the 1987 redefinition, is problematic in its impact on statistics and needs estimates but even more in its impact on individuals affected, because the CDC definition is used in eligibility determinations for health and income maintenance benefits.

Persons with HIV illness who have not attained the CDC criterion receive separate and unequal treatment in qualifying for public health care and financial benefits (Crystal and Jackson 1988). Unlike those with AIDS (who suffer from one of the presumptively disabling conditions listed on the Social Security Administrations's "Disability Report" Form 3368), they are not presumed to be disabled for purposes of benefits determination but are subject to a lengthy case-by-case determination of disability, a process that sometimes lasts longer than the benefit applicant. Social Security Administration benefits like Social Security Disability Insurance payments (SSDI) and Supplemental Security Income (SSI) are crucial for persons who are suffering from the debilitating and disabling effects of the infection. Medicaid, another crucial benefit, is also tied to the disability determination process; for example, it typically is provided automatically to SSI recipients. At the end of the labyrinth, those with HIV illness but not AIDS may or may not ultimately succeed in gaining access to these basic survival benefits, even though, as the data that follow suggest, they often are unable to work and are certainly likely to need costly medical care.

Thus, with HIV as with other types of illness, our unique U.S. approach to health care financing creates separate classes of ill people. One such class has access through medicare to publicly financed benefits without means testing. This class includes the elderly and also the severely disabled, but the latter are subject to a 2-year waiting period, barring most AIDS patients from eligibility. Another class, presumedly disabled, is eligible for income benefits (SSDI or SSI) and, by virtue of disability, is eligible for medicaid on a means-tested basis but not for medicare. A third category is likely to have difficulty accessing even means-tested benefits. The elderly and long-term disabled are thus defined, de facto, as medically deserving; other disabled are assigned to the limbo of conditional deservingness (provided they impoverish themselves first); and the third group, if not privately insured, enter the purgatory of "self-pay" or become part of a hospital's bad debt. Those not "officially" disabled and without health coverage are likely to experience increased frustration in their attempts to secure needed medical care.

Experience with the health care system for persons with HIV infection but not AIDS is shaped by these definitions and by the concomitant fact that many of their most disabling symptoms are nonspecific ones. A specific condition such as Kaposi's sarcoma establishes clear-cut eligibility for benefits but may not in itself be particularly impairing. Persons with ARC, although lacking such defining conditions, are likely to suffer from such conditions as chronic and debilitating fatigue, night sweats, diarrhea, headaches, sleep loss, and inability to concentrate. Such conditions can be chronic, recurring, and thoroughly incapacitating but are likely to be unpersuasive to a disability examiner and may not be responded to as urgently, or taken as seriously, by medical personnel.

The use of the CDC AIDS definition in benefit eligibility reflects an implicit assumption that, because patients with AIDS-related complex are at an earlier stage, medically, of the progression of the HIV infection, the disabling effects of the disease and the care needs created by it are less severe. To evaluate this assumption and to compare the experience of persons with differently defined HIV illness, two surveys of persons with differently defined HIV-related conditions were conducted in San Diego County, California.

METHODS AND FINDINGS

The first of the two surveys (late 1986 and early 1987) preceded the September 1987 CDC definition change. We included both persons with AIDS and with what, at that time, was generally referred to as AIDS-related complex, or ARC. The survey was intended to ascertain medical, social, economic, and other needs and the way they were being met. We included persons with ARC as well as those with AIDS because less attention has been paid to their needs, and designed the survey to permit comparisons between the two groups. Data were collected on 50 persons with AIDS (PWAs) and 54 persons with ARC (PWARCs) at diverse sites to maximize sample diversity and minimize bias. Questionnaires were distributed by staff members at health care sites across the county (n = 48) and at support groups and social events for PWAs/PWARCs (n = 29); 27 interviews were conducted by a medical student at a university medical center outpatient HIV clinic site.

A second survey (n = 324) was conducted from December 1989 through January 1990. Three categories of self-assignment were used; those who had been told they had AIDS (PWAs); those who had been told they had AIDS-related complex (PWARCs); and those with a positive antibody test to HIV (PWHIVs). Although not always consistently used as a medical term, it was found that *ARC* remained a meaningful term commonly used by medical providers and patients to characterize symptomatic HIV illness that did not attain the CDC criterion for AIDS. We included seropositive persons (PWHIVs) to determine how their needs differed from those reported by persons with more severe illness. In addition, we wanted to develop information on reported use of community-based organizations that provide a variety of services in order to provide information that could be used by these organizations when seeking funding from private and public sources. Survey instruments were distributed through staff at major health care and social service sites across the county; a medical student also recruited and assisted subjects at the county's AIDS Assistance Fund, which provides assistance with food, clothing, and shelter.

1986-87 Survey

The 1986-87 survey instrument covered a range of areas including demographic characteristics, social supports, economic situation, and health services use. Five-point Likert-type scales were developed to assess the extent to which medical and socioeconomic needs of patients were being met in areas such as income, access to outpatient and inpatient care, social services assistance, relief for persons providing care, psychological counseling, household help, and so on. Additional series of scales assessed social support, the response of persons in the patient's social network to the illness, and satisfaction with various aspects of available medical care. The 104 respondents also were asked about the social and economic consequences of their illness and about the medical symptoms they had experienced. (Survey methods and findings are discussed in greater detail in Crystal and Jackson 1989.)

Many, but by no means all, of the respondents who were no longer employed received disability or welfare benefits: 84% of nonemployed AIDS patients, but only 41% of those with ARC, relied on Supplemental Security Income (SSI) and/or social security disability benefits. Many of those with AIDS-related complex relied on local general assistance welfare payments, savings, family, or a lover; the proportion of nonemployed ARC patients who relied on these sources or who had no income was 41%. These results appear to reflect the easier access to benefits associated with a diagnosis of CDC-defined "AIDS." Eligibility for income benefits has important implications for health benefits eligibility. SSI eligibility brings with it eligibility for medicaid in most states, including California, whereas, in California, those dependent on local general assistance programs receive financial benefits considerably lower than those provided by SSI and are not eligible for Medicaid.

As a result of loss of employment and relatively low or nonexistent benefit payments in many cases, survey respondents had typically suffered dramatic income declines since diagnosis. Mean income at the time of survey completion was $11,800, or 58% of prediagnosis income. The majority (69%) had incomes under $10,000. When asked about their greatest unmet area of need for help, the most frequent response both for persons with AIDS and for those with AIDS-related complex was "financial."

In addition to the income loss, patients had typically suffered a number of other negative socioeconomic consequences of the disease. Almost half (46%) had been unable to pay for needed medical care; this was true of nearly two thirds of the ARC patients (64%) and of nearly one third of the AIDS patients (29%). Difficulty in keeping up with household chores was an even more prevalent problem, affecting 70% of ARC patients and 47%

of AIDS patients. AIDS patients were more likely to be eligible for entitlements that brought with them access to home care services but still did not have all their needs met in this area. The greater unmet need for help with homemaking chores experienced by persons with ARC may be because PWARCs are less likely to have access to entitlement programs providing homemaker assistance. Without special funding streams for PWARCs, their situation could become even worse as the numbers increase and as the homemaker assistance resources of charitable and voluntary organizations are exhausted attempting to meet the needs of persons with AIDS.

For the sample as a whole, other socioeconomic problems encountered included loss of a job due to health problems (50%), loss of a job due to fear or discrimination (19%), loss of friends due to fear (41%), loss of housing due to fear or discrimination (13%), loss of housing because of the loss of income (21%), rejection by some family members (34%), and difficulty with transportation (34%). Of 11 such areas about which respondents were questioned, ARC patients had encountered problems more frequently in 8 of the areas, often by wide margins, whereas AIDS patients had experienced problems more frequently in 3 areas. The difference was highly significant (p < .01 by chi-square) for inability to pay for medical care but did not attain statistical significance in the other areas.

Although persons with AIDS-related complex suffered from conditions usually considered to be less severe than those with AIDS, and are believed to have a less uniformly grave prognosis, they typically had been ill for a longer period. Most of the PWAs had been diagnosed within the previous year; only 9 (18%) had been diagnosed prior to 1986. The majority had not received a diagnosis of ARC prior to being diagnosed with AIDS; only 11 of the 50 PWAs reported being diagnosed with ARC prior to an AIDS diagnosis. Where possible, PWAs were recontacted to confirm the absence of a previous ARC diagnosis. PWARCs typically had lived with a diagnosed HIV-related condition for considerably longer than PWAs. A majority (59%) had been diagnosed prior to 1986, and almost a quarter (22%) had been diagnosed prior to 1985, with diagnosis dates stretching back as far as 1981. Mean time since the first ARC or AIDS diagnosis for PWAs (N = 50) was 9.2 months, and mean time since diagnosis for the PWARCs (N = 53) was 14.7 months. For the 11 persons diagnosed first with ARC, the mean time interval from ARC to AIDS diagnosis was 9.82 months. The overall mean time interval from diagnosis of AIDS or ARC to the time the survey was completed by all respondents (N = 103) was about one year (mean = 11.99 months). Thus, on average, those with ARC had been suffering from symptomatic disease for about half again as long as those with AIDS and had a longer period during which financial, emotional, or social resources might be exhausted.

When respondents were asked to volunteer additional symptoms not mentioned on the checklist, 24% of PWARCs, compared with none of the PWAs, mentioned "fatigue" specifically. When asked how HIV-related medical problems had limited usual activities, about 80% of PWARCs and 74% of PWAs responded that the lethargy or fatigue interfered with daily activities. Those with AIDS-related complex were more likely to report having their activities limited by pain or by decreased concentration than those with AIDS and were more likely to have suffered night sweats, severe diarrhea, or headaches. This pattern of complaints suggests that those with ARC reported at least as significant "quality of life" symptoms as those with AIDS, although *acute* illness, as indicated by hospitalization histories, had been more typical of the PWAs. Over 75% of PWAs reported one or more episodes of hospitalization since diagnosis compared with only 37% of PWARCs, and 47% of PWAs versus 17% of PWARCs had been hospitalized for a total of more than 9 days since diagnosis.

A number of areas of need were listed on the questionnaire. Respondents were asked to rate, using a Likert-type scale (1 = *not at all met*; 5 = *very adequately met*), how well each listed need was met. The proportion of persons reporting unmet needs was higher for those with ARC than for those with AIDS in 14 of 16 need areas asked about, with the difference statistically significant (p < .05) in 4 of the areas; neither of the two differences in the other direction was statistically significant. In addition, a mean need satisfaction score was calculated for each area of need for PWA and PWARC respondents. Again, PWARCs indicated that their needs were being less than adequately met (represented by a mean score below 3.0) in more than half of the areas of need, whereas mean scores for PWAs were less than 3.0 in only two areas of need. Mean need satisfaction score was lower for PWARCs than for PWAs in 14 of the 16 areas (significantly so in 4 areas) and higher for PWARCs in only 2 areas (significantly so in 1 of the 2). When data for respondents from both groups were combined, the greatest unmet need was clearly for income.

1989-90 Survey

In the 1989-90 survey, 324 respondents were asked to indicate the most likely route of exposure to HIV: 85% of the respondents indicted sexual exposure, with an additional 10% (32) indicating "don't know" or a combination of risk behaviors. Only 11 persons circled intravenous (IV) drug use as the only risk behavior; 6 persons indicated blood products as the exposure route. As with the first survey, the survey findings principally describe the circumstances of a predominantly white, male homosexual population. San Diego County surveillance data indicate that this characterizes the county population of PWAs as a whole. Of reported AIDS cases through July 31, 1990, 80% were white non-Hispanic, and 96% were men. Only 5% were attributed to IV drug use alone and another 7% reported both IV drug use and male homosexual/bisexual risk behaviors (San Diego County Department of Health Services 1990). In addition, the minority of people of color were underrepresented in the survey in all three diagnostic groups when compared with the country surveillance data and with data on persons who have been found to be HIV-antibody positive at the San Diego County Department of Health Services Alternative Test Sites (ATS). In the survey, only 20 respondents indicated they were of color (7 blacks and 13 Hispanics). We believe this underrepresentation may relate to the geographic distribution of participating agencies in the downtown San Diego area and to the fact that many persons of color may be particularly suspicious of a survey sponsored by an arm of a government agency (the San Diego Country Regional Task Force on AIDS).

Educational status was similar to that in the 1986-87 survey: About 80% of all respondents had some college and many had college degrees. Monthly income was variable by group, with higher incomes reported by a larger proportion of seropositives (PWHIVs) and lower incomes reported by PWAs. In fact, about 65% of PWAs, 61% of PWARCs, and 32% of PWHIVs reported monthly incomes of less than $1,000. In this respect, PWARCs appeared more like PWAs than like PWHIVs.

Employment status also varied by group, with 82% of those with AIDS, 56% of those with ARC, and 35% of seropositives reporting that they were not employed. Of persons unemployed, 75% of those with AIDS, 57% of those with ARC, and 25% of the PWHIVs received social security (SSI or SSDI) benefits. Of the total group, 26% of PWAs, 11% of PWARCs, and 11% of PWHIVs received state disability; 5% of those with AIDS, and none of the PWARCs or PWHIVs, received Veterans Administration or military benefits.

With better access to disability benefits, the PWAs apparently had less need for the much less generous General Relief benefits, because only 2% used these benefits, versus 6% of the PWARCs and 10% of the PWHIVs. It is important that those with ARC were much less likely to qualify for health benefits through Medicare, Medicaid, or military programs: 49% of those with AIDS received Medicaid versus 26% of those with ARC and none of the seropositives; 11% of the PWAs received Medicare versus 8% of PWARCs and only 1 of the 110 PWHIVs.

An important finding of this survey was derived from the list of symptoms selected by the persons in each category. Of interest, only 20% of the seropositives reported symptoms such as fever/chills, herpes infection, skin infections, and severe fatigue. Although substantially fewer PWHIVs reported these symptoms than did PWARCs and PWAs, these symptoms are associated with sufficient functional impairment that some physicians would classify the person as a PWARC. It is possible that some of the "PWHIVs" may be denying their more severe diagnoses. The possible presence of functional impairment among some defining themselves as "persons with HIV" may also help explain why 35% of the PWHIVs reported they were not employed and, of those not employed, several were receiving either SSI/SSDI or state disability. On the other hand, 5 (18%) of the unemployed PWHIVs reported receiving a pension (including military) and may have been unemployed due to retirement. Because the survey relied on self-report for diagnostic classification—respondents were reporting what they had been told they had, or understood themselves to have, rather than direct diagnostic information having been received from medical providers—some respondents may have reported a diagnostic classification different than that which would have been produced by a review of medical data. However, just as relevant as the biological facts in each case may be the category that the individual and relevant others assume to apply.

Between the first and second surveys, the September 1987 redefinition and broadening of the CDC AIDS definition took place. After the redefinition, some (but not all) persons with symptomatic HIV illness, who would previously have been labeled as cases of AIDS-related complex, would instead be classified into the AIDS category. (Cases of HIV-induced wasting syndrome, for example, were an important category added to the AIDS definition at that time.) One might expect that a postredefinition survey of persons with HIV illness in a community would identify a somewhat smaller number of persons with AIDS-related complex (especially those with severe symptomatology) as compared with those with AIDS. This is consistent with the observation that only 29% of the combined AIDS and ARC cases in the second survey fell into the ARC category (54 ARC and 50 AIDS in the first survey, 62 ARC and 152 AIDS in the second). In addition, a significantly smaller proportion of PWARCs in the second survey reported unexplained weight loss (67% in the first survey as compared with 30% in the second survey; $p < .001$). This may reflect the inclusion of wasting syndrome in the AIDS case definition. Comparisons between the two surveys are also possible for four other symptoms, with a nonsignificant decline for severe diarrhea (37% versus 54%), night sweats (68% versus 83%), and lymphadenopathy (52% versus 65%), and a nonsignificant increase for candida (73% versus 61%).

Results of a comparison of the responses to needs assessment items provided by persons with AIDS and those with ARC on the second survey also are consistent with the presumption that more of those with severe HIV illness were being categorized as having AIDS rather than ARC by 1989-90. Such needs as in-home care provision and relief of caregivers were more likely in the second survey to be checked off as "inapplicable." Need satisfaction scores in the second survey for those with AIDS and for those with ARC were quite similar in most domains. In contrast with the first survey—and despite the larger sample size—none of the differences in any of the 22 need categories was statistically significant.

The pattern of similarity suggests that the socioeconomic, psychological, and functional impacts of disease on the group still labeled as "ARC" cases continued to be severe. In the important domain of income, for example, 46% reported needs inadequately met, similar to the proportion of 48% for those with AIDS; and 45% reported needs inadequately met for dental care, 27% for outpatient medical care, 34% for psychological counseling, and 34% in the area of spiritual needs. (Results for those with AIDS were 45%, 18%, 34%, and 23% respectively). Although those in the "ARC" category in 1989-90 no longer tended to perceive themselves as doing *worse* than those with AIDS, they still did not report themselves as doing *better,* even though severe symptomatology had decreased somewhat. Thus a presumption that the medically less "severe" condition had less severe impact would not be supported by these observations. As with PWAs, a majority were unable to work for medical or other reasons; income inadequacy was widespread; and rates of unmet needs were generally comparable to those of the respondents with full-blown AIDS.

DISCUSSION

As compared with the rest of the nation, San Diego County's population of PWAs and PWARCs contains relatively fewer persons with social histories of poverty, poor education, and other indicators that would suggest a lack of personal, economic, and social resources. Even though PWAs and PWARCs in San Diego tend to have high levels of education and relatively high prediagnosis occupational status and income, they were overwhelmed by the disabling impact of the disease, and their social and economic resources were typically unable to meet the needs precipitated by their illness. In both surveys, most persons with AIDS and a majority of those with ARC were no longer able to be employed. PWARCs, in particular, were likely to have no health coverage at all. In the 1986-87 survey, only 13% of PWARCs received Medicaid despite their typically very low or nonexistent incomes; this proportion had doubled (26%) by 1989-90 but was still quite low. The result was an inability to meet many basic needs of everyday life as well as to pay for medical care. In the group surveyed in 1986-87, nearly two thirds of PWARCs had been unable to pay for needed medical care (this question was not asked in the same way in 1989-90).

Although the results of both surveys may not be entirely representative of all PWAs in the area at the time, it is apparent that the problems experienced by PWAs continue to be quite serious and will undoubtedly get worse as the numbers increase. The needs of the PWA population in San Diego and areas like it, although not of the magnitude of those in New York, San Francisco, or Los Angeles, will increasingly strain health care and social services systems.

In addition to the better publicized needs of PWAs, the surveys identified the severe nature of the unmet needs of the larger population of PWARCs. Even after the reclassification, unmet needs of PWARCs were comparable to those of PWAs, even though the former had not experienced bouts of pneumocystis pneumonia or other AIDS-defining events and were less likely to have required hospitalization. This appears to be the result of the longer period of illness experienced by PWARCs, who often had exhausted their resources, and their greater difficulty in quali-fying for public benefits such as social security disability, Supplemental Security Income, and Medicaid, which have used a diagnosis of AIDS, but not of ARC, as presumptive proof of disability. Medicaid in particular is crucial because, as a result of the 2-year waiting period, few in either the PWA or the PWARC category can benefit from medicare benefits available to other disabled individuals.

One major need identified by PWAs and PWARCs in the first survey was for medical care that was not only technically good but accessible and perceived as well coordinated, available in emergencies, caring, and with good communication among patients, their significant others, and the care providers. By the time of the second survey, a much larger network of care providers was available in San Diego as were four different "Case Management Programs" (provided by the Visiting Nurses Association, the County Department of Health Services, the Veterans Administration Medical Center, and the Area Agency on Aging) to coor-dinate care. Unfortunately, funding for these programs has been fragile, and continued funding is quite uncertain. The economic crisis for PWARCs and PWAs is becoming an even more urgent issue as costly medications like AZT come into wider use. Funding for these medications for persons without third party coverage for their costs through medicaid or health insurance also has been erratic, with "temporary" programs put in place without a stable funding stream.

Persons with ARC have been characterized as living in a "limbo of Hell," and comments to this effect have been made when results of this survey were discussed with other researchers and with PWARCs and PWAs. Their situation has been described by one patient as "life in the gray zone" (Morin, Charles, and Malyon 1984). Once a person meets CDC criteria for a diagnosis of AIDS, there is some certainty about the future. Although, currently, a diagnosis of AIDS typically implies that death from the disease is likely within 2 to 4 years, it also means automatic entitlement to various programs that make meeting daily activities of living somewhat easier. The process of coping psychologically with this terminal diagnosis is, of course, extremely stressful. As with cancer and other catastrophic or terminal diagnoses (Weisman 1979), psycho-social adaptation as the physical disease evolves has been discussed in terms of a multistage reaction process, with progression from initial shock through anger and denial to ultimate acceptance and preparation for dying (Forstein, 1984; Nichols 1985; Wolcott 1986). The uncertainty of an

AIDS-related complex diagnosis, however, may be even more stressful, with great anxiety surrounding each new symptom. Symptoms particularly characteristic of ARC, such as very severe chronic diarrhea, extreme fatigue, and night sweats, can be devastatingly disabling (Volberding 1985) while not engendering the same degree of attention by medical providers as may more specific conditions accompanying AIDS.

Kaplan, Johnson, Bailey, and Simon (1989) model the degree of subjective distress caused by AIDS-related stress as a function of the value placed on health status, life-style, specific behavior patterns, acceptance by others, personal and interpersonal resources that are threatened, and the general ability to assuage distress, which, in turn, is a function of such variables as beliefs about self-efficacy and normal adaptive, coping, and defensive patterns. To this list should be added the way in which uncertainty is managed. In one of the still relatively few sociological studies of the experience of living with HIV, Weitz (1989) reported on findings from a sample of 23 men self-reporting with AIDS or ARC. Although this report, with its small sample, was unable to compare the experiences of the two groups, it strongly illuminated the role of uncertainty as a central, and profoundly distressing, experience in the lives of persons with HIV disease. Because those who are symptomatic but not yet diagnosed with "official" AIDS are in a particularly uncertain situation, it may well be the case that the dilemmas of uncertainty are even more severe and anxiety provoking.

Because of limited resources among care providers, persons with AIDS may be able to access the health care system with greater ease because their symptoms may be viewed as more serious and in need of more immediate intervention. For example, treatment for pneumocystis pneumonia is most effective if begun early, and it receives a high priority for medical care. Medical care can be more difficult for PWARCs to obtain, and this pattern appears anecdotally to be true even where service availability is relatively good. In San Francisco, for example, the presence has been noted of "a great many people with ARC who have debilitating conditions and need all the services we can provide, yet some of them may not qualify for services because they do not have the strict AIDS clinical diagnosis, as defined by the Centers for Disease Control" (Silverman 1987). ARC often progresses to AIDS but frequently is a cause of long-term and severely disabling morbidity without progressing to AIDS and can be a cause of death even without such progression, even after the 1987 definition change.

Few survey data are yet available on the adequacy with which economic, medical, and other needs of daily life of PWAs and PWARCs are met. One study reported in 1985 did suggest that PWARCs may manifest more psychological distress than those with the full-blown disease (Tross 1985). Our findings support the view that coping with ARC can be just as difficult as or more difficult than coping with AIDS. Further, the results of the 1989-90 survey indicate that, even after the 1987 redefinition, there remain a group of individuals with severely impairing symptomatology and major health care needs who fall short of the official CDC AIDS definition. The continued use of that definition, constructed for epidemiological and surveillance purposes, in disability determination and by benefits systems continues to impose a medically somewhat arbitrary distinction between often similarly situated individuals, substantially affecting many aspects of their experience with the illness.

Persons with ARC generally manifest symptoms that are less specific than those of PWAs; many of these symptoms do not respond well to medical treatment. In addition, because of the uncertainties associated with a diagnosis of ARC, the individual is often unsure of the significance of symptoms and uncertain whether the current illness will "make criteria for AIDS" or not. Thus contact with health care providers may occur often due to anxiety but may be met with a perceived lack of responsiveness or inadequate communication by medical providers.

Individuals with significant symptomatology, whether referred to as cases of AIDS, ARC, "associated opportunistic infections," or other terminology, in turn, represent only part of the population of persons infected with the human immunodeficiency virus. As more infected persons become symptomatic, resource and service needs will continue to increase. The magnitude of health care needs is understated by reliance on statistics reflecting only those with "official" AIDS. This highlights the need to develop new financing mechanisms to meet care needs for persons at all points in the spectrum of HIV illness, including individuals, largely asymptomatic, with HIV infection who can benefit from early intervention with AZT, pentamidine, or other medication but who may not have the financial wherewithal to pay for preventive treatment.

Indeed, the use of the term *AIDS* as shorthand for the epidemic of HIV illness represents a semantic lag carried over from the era preceding knowledge of the cause of the illness. Today, the construction of the epidemic as the "AIDS problem" rather than the "HIV illness problem" subtly biases our thinking about the nature of the challenge and focuses attention away from the very real problems of the larger HIV-infected population and toward a smaller population of late-stage cases. Although there is an increasing trend among medical and research personnel to speak of HIV illness rather than AIDS, this shift is by no means systematic and the epidemic is still almost always spoken of in common parlance as the "AIDS epidemic." The slowness of change in the language used contrasts sharply with the very rapid semantic shift that took place earlier in the epidemic, when the earlier-used labels coined by competing teams of researchers (HTLV-III by American labs and LAV by the French) were replaced by "HIV," a term not previously identified with either group. Where scientific credit and national prestige were at stake, semantic issues took on special salience for medical researchers, but the effects of the AIDS synecdoche appear to lack similar salience.

Persons with HIV infection themselves have been among those most acutely aware of the political and practical implications of language. Thus, for example, the tendency of the media to refer to "AIDS victims" has been strongly resisted by persons with AIDS or HIV infection, as casting them in a preconceived victim role. Similarly, the term *intravenous drug abuser,* with its pejorative connotations, has been largely replaced by intravenous *drug user* and, more recently in some quarters, by *injection drug user* (because not all persons at risk through needle sharing use needles intravenously). But the misleading semantic implications of talking about AIDS when we mean the HIV epidemic, talking about persons with AIDS when we mean the HIV infected, and talking about AIDS health care when we mean HIV health care are continuing to shape the way in which the epidemic is seen and in which the policy issues are framed. This is particularly the case because the distribution of cases of full-blown AIDS represents the past of the epidemic, not its present and certainly not its future. Refocusing both our language and our policies on the broader problem of HIV infection is more than just a matter of semantic clarity. It is part of the reorientation, or paradigm shift, that is needed from an acute disease to a chronic disease model; from a focus on end-stage disease to an emphasis on the continuum of illness and on early intervention; and from thinking in terms of the persons dying with AIDS in favor of a focus on what is needed by those who are living with HIV.

REFERENCES

Brandt, Allan. 1985. *No Magic Bullet: A Social History of Venereal Disease in the United States Since 1880.* New York: Oxford University Press.

Cowie, Bill. 1976. "The Cardiac Patient's Perception of His Heart Attack." *Social Science and Medicine* 10:87-96.

Crystal, Stephen and Marguerite Jackson. 1988. "The Hidden Epidemic: AIDS-Related Complex: Living in the Gray Zone." *AIDS Patient Care* 2(4):4-7.

————. 1989. "Psychosocial Adaptation and Economic Circumstances of Persons With AIDS and AIDS-Related Complex." *Family and Community Health* 12(2):77-88.

Forstein, Marshall. 1984. "The Psychosocial Impact of the Acquired Immunodeficiency Syndrome." *Seminars in Oncology* 11(1):77-82.

Gilman, Sander L. 1988. *Disease and Representation: Images of Illness From Madness to AIDS.* Ithaca, NY: Cornell University Press.

Institute of Medicine. 1986. *Confronting AIDS: Directions for Public Health, Health Care, and Research.* Washington, DC: National Academy Press.

————. 1988. *Confronting AIDS: Update 1988.* Washington, DC: National Academy Press.

Kaplan, Howard B., Robert J. Johnson, Carol A. Bailey, and William Simon. 1989. "The Sociological Study of AIDS: A Critical Review of the Literature and Suggested Research Agenda." *Journal of Health and Social Behavior* 28:140-57.

McKinlay, John B., Katherine Skinner, John W. Riley, Jr., and Diane Zablotsky. 1989. "On the Relevance of Social Science Concepts and Perspectives." Pp. 127-46 in *AIDS in an Aging Society: What We Need to Know,* edited by M. W. Riley, M. G. Ory, and D. Zablotsky. New York: Springer.

Mechanic, David. 1978. *Medical Sociology.* 2nd ed. New York: Free Press.

Morin, Stephen F., Kenneth A. Charles, and Alan K. Malyon. 1984. "The Psychological Impact of AIDS on Gay Men." *American Psychologist* 39:1288-93.

Nichols, Stuart E. 1985. "Psychosocial Reactions of Persons With the Acquired Immuno-deficiency Syndrome." *Annals of Internal Medicine* 103:765-67.

Oppenheimer, Gerald M. 1988. "In the Eye of the Storm: The Epidemiological Construction of AIDS." Pp. 267-300 in *AIDS: The Burdens of History,* edited by E. Fee and D. M. Fox. Berkeley: University of California Press.

Rosenberg, Charles E. 1988. "Disease and Social Order in America: Perceptions and Expectations." Pp. 12-32 in *AIDS: The Burdens of History,* edited by E. Fee and D. M. Fox. Berkeley: University of California Press.

San Diego County Department of Health Services. 1990. *San Diego County Reported Resident Cases of AIDS, Monthly Surveillance Report* (July 31). San Diego, CA: Author.

Schneider, Joseph W. and Peter Conrad. 1983. *Having Epilepsy: The Experience and Control of Illness.* Philadelphia: Temple University Press.

Silverman, Mervyn. 1987. "San Francisco: Coordinated Community Response." Pp. 170-81 in *AIDS: Public Policy Dimensions,* edited by J. Griggs. New York: United Hospital Fund.

Sontag, Susan. 1989. *AIDS and Its Metaphors.* New York: Farrar, Straus, and Giroux.

Tross, Susan. 1985. "Psychological and Neuropsychological Functions in AIDS Patients."
    Presented to the International Conference on AIDS.
Volberding, Paul A. 1985. "The Clinical Spectrum of the Acquired Immunodeficiency
    Syndrome: Implications for Comprehensive Patient Care." *Annals of Internal Medi-
    cine* 103:729-33.
Weisman, Avery D. 1979. "A Model for Psychosocial Staging in Cancer." *General Hospital
    Psychiatry* 1:187-95.
Weitz, Rose. 1989. "Uncertainty and the Lives of Persons With AIDS." *Journal of Health
    and Social Behavior* 30:270-81.
Wolcott, Deane L. 1986. "Psychosocial Aspects of Acquired Immune Deficiency Syndrome
    and the Primary Care Physician." *Annals of Allergy* 57:95-102.

Glossary

AIDS (acquired immune deficiency syndrome). Name applied to a clinical syndrome identified by medical doctors early in the 1980s to connote an acquired disease, one that could be passed from person to person, and a set of symptoms reflecting a defect in the body's immune system. In the most popular classification of the disease, AIDS is considered the full-blown syndrome, the most severe manifestation of infection with human immunodeficiency virus, which destroys important components of the human immune system. Persons with the disease develop infections that would not occur with normal immunity. Death in persons with AIDS is due primarily to a variety of different opportunistic diseases and associated conditions, not directly to HIV infection itself. The Centers for Disease Control have strict criteria for a diagnosis of AIDS, which is similar to full-blown AIDS in the popular classification. The term *AIDS* has become part of the common language typically used by most people and the media to talk about this illness, as in "AIDS crisis" or "AIDS epidemic."

ARC (AIDS-related complex). A variety of chronic symptoms and physical findings that occur in some persons who are infected with HIV but whose conditions do not meet the Centers for Disease Control definition of AIDS. Symptoms may include persistent swollen lymph nodes, recurrent fevers, unintentional weight loss, chronic diarrhea, lethargy, and minor alterations of the immune system. ARC may or may not develop into AIDS.

AZT (Azidothymidine). Main drug used to prevent the further replication of the human immunodeficiency virus. It does not kill the virus but halts viral replication. Those medically able to take AZT typically take it for the remainder of their lives. AZT seems to prolong the lives of PWAs and PWARCs, primarily by boosting their level of immune system functioning. AZT is the only drug fully tested and approved by the U.S. government for treatment of persons with AIDS.

CDC (Centers for Disease Control). U.S. government agency that performs epidemiological study and surveillance of disease, mortality, and morbidity and develops and conducts programs for disease prevention. The CDC surveillance definition of AIDS can be understood as the legal definition of AIDS, the one used for enumeration of reported AIDS cases in the United States and for determination of eligibility for welfare and health benefits.

HIV (human immunodeficiency virus). Internationally agreed-upon label for the virus understood to be the cause of immune system failure resulting, in many cases, in AIDS. Prior to this designation by the International Subcommittee on the Taxonomy of Virus, it was known as HTLV-III, or human T-cell lymphotropic virus type III, by National Cancer Institute researchers in the United States, and as LAV, or lymphadenopathy-associated virus, by researchers in France.

HIV infection (or HIV disease). Used to describe the full spectrum of infection by human immunodeficiency virus from an asymptomatic carrier, a person who is infected but feels or shows no outward symptoms, to a person with a diagnosed case of AIDS.

IVDU (intravenous drug user). Person who uses intravenous needles to inject illegal drugs, such as heroin or cocaine, into his or her body. Intravenous means "inserted into the vein." IV needles and syringes (the plastic container attached to the IV needle) are both transmitters of HIV. The virus is transmitted through blood that remains in the needle or syringe after injection, not through the injected drug itself.

PWA (person with AIDS). Identity label developed by people who were suffering from complications of AIDS to destigmatize two of the metaphors used to characterize AIDS, the metaphors of death and punishment, which found their way into everyday discourse in terms such as "AIDS victim," "invariably fatal," "promiscuous," "AIDS patient," and "innocent victim." This redefinition process was a means by which an emphasis could be put on processes of living and dying, with dignity and without blame, and on a person's ability to take control of his or her life. The initials were picked up by others; PWARC and PWHIV have been used as abbreviations, respectively, for persons with AIDS-related complex and persons with HIV infection.

Index